Anti-Inflammatory Diet Cookbook for Beginners 2024

Easy and Healthy Meals to Enhance Immunity and Reduce Chronic Pain

Dr. Donald M. Dermers

Table of Content

Introduction

In the haste and bustle of modern life, keeping a healthy lifestyle can be a strain. However, knowing the wonderful power of 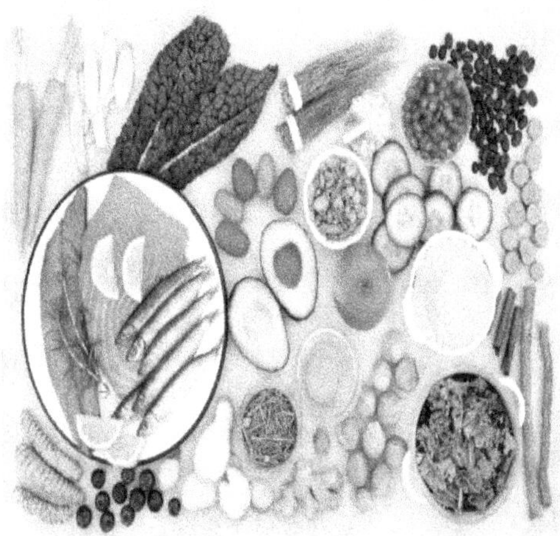 food as medicine is a vital step towards achieving optimal well-being.

In this cookbook, we embark on a journey to demystify the anti-inflammatory diet, offering you accessible, delicious, and beginner-friendly recipes that empower you to take care of your health.

Inflammation, typically the fundamental cause of various chronic diseases, is significantly influenced by the foods we consume. This cookbook serves as your guide to embracing an anti-inflammatory lifestyle, featuring a varied range of nutrient-dense meals carefully created for beginners. Whether you're aiming to prevent diseases or simply increase your general health, these recipes are designed to make the shift to an anti-inflammatory diet smooth and pleasurable.

Within these pages, you'll discover the foundations of anti-inflammatory eating, learn how to stock your kitchen with necessary products and master the art of meal planning and preparation. The aim of this guide is to not only supply you with tasty recipes but also to empower you with the knowledge to make informed choices about the foods you consume.

Embark on this gastronomic trip and discover the transformational impact of anti-inflammatory eating. Let this cookbook be your companion on the way to a healthier, more vibrant you. Welcome to a world where food is not only a source of enjoyment but also a strong tool for fostering wellness. Let's cook our way to a life of vigor and longevity together!

Understanding Inflammation:

Inflammation is a natural and vital aspect of the body's immunological response. It is the method the body fights itself against damaging stimuli, such as diseases, injuries, or toxins. The process involves the activation of the immune system, resulting in the production of numerous substances that work to eliminate the cause of cell harm, clear out damaged cells, and commence tissue repair.

The two different types of inflammation: are acute and chronic. Acute inflammation is a short-term and localized response to an injury or infection, while chronic inflammation persists over a longer period and is typically connected with many health issues, including autoimmune illnesses and chronic diseases.

Understanding inflammation entails recognizing the signs and symptoms, such as redness, swelling, pain, and loss of function. It is vital to differentiate between acute and chronic inflammation, as chronic inflammation can lead to the development of numerous diseases.

Nutrition plays a vital function in controlling the inflammatory response in the body. Certain foods can either stimulate or reduce inflammation. A diet rich in anti-inflammatory foods can help reduce chronic inflammation and improve general health. Key components in this context include:

- Omega-3 Fatty Acids: Found in fatty fish (such as salmon and mackerel), flaxseeds, chia seeds, and walnuts, omega-3 fatty acids offer anti-inflammatory qualities.

- Antioxidants: Fruits and vegetables are abundant in antioxidants, which help counteract oxidative stress and inflammation. Berries, leafy greens, and colored veggies are excellent sources.

- Whole Grains: Foods like brown rice, quinoa, and oats give fiber and nutrients that contribute to a healthy inflammatory response.

- Spices and Herbs: Turmeric, ginger, garlic, and cinnamon are examples of culinary herbs and spices that offer anti-inflammatory qualities.

- Probiotics: Found in fermented foods like yogurt, kefir, and sauerkraut, probiotics enhance intestinal health, impacting the body's inflammatory response.

Fruits and Vegetables:

- ★ They help counteract oxidative stress and inflammation, boosting general health. Aim for a colorful selection to optimize nutritional advantages.
- ★ Rich in vitamins, minerals, fiber, and antioxidants, fruits and vegetables are vital components of an anti-inflammatory diet.

Whole Grains:

- ★ Whole grains, such as brown rice, quinoa, oats, and whole wheat, provide complex carbs, fiber, and different nutrients. They help to steady blood sugar levels and have anti-inflammatory qualities, boosting overall well-being.

Healthy Fats:

★ Omega-3 fatty acids found in fatty fish (salmon, mackerel), flaxseeds, chia seeds, and walnuts are anti-inflammatory fats. Additionally, monounsaturated fats from sources like olive oil and avocados can help control inflammation and enhance heart health.

Lean Proteins:

★ Choose lean protein sources such as poultry, fish, lentils, and tofu. These options supply necessary amino acids without the saturated fats frequently found in red and processed meats, which can lead to inflammation.

★ Herbs and spices including turmeric, ginger, garlic, cinnamon, and basil contain bioactive components with anti-inflammatory properties. Incorporating these into your meals provides taste while encouraging health.

★ Opt for cooking methods including sautéing, roasting, and steaming. These strategies retain the nutritional content of foods and can boost the anti-inflammatory benefits of your meals.

A well-stocked pantry is the basis of a healthy kitchen. Include:

- Whole Grains: Brown rice, quinoa, oats.
- Healthy Fats: Olive oil, avocados, nuts, and seeds.
- Legumes: Beans, lentils, chickpeas.
- Herbs and Spices: Turmeric, ginger, garlic, cinnamon, basil.
- Canned Tomatoes: A source of lycopene, recognized for its anti-inflammatory qualities.

Equip your kitchen with items that make making anti-inflammatory meals convenient:

- Quality Knives: For chopping fruits, vegetables, and lean proteins.

- Cutting Boards: Use different boards for meats and produce.

- Blender or Food Processor: Great for smoothies, sauces, and homemade dressings.

- Steamer Basket: Preserves nutrients in veggies throughout cooking.

- Non-Stick Pans: Reduce the need for unnecessary cooking oils.

- Baking Sheets and Cooking Pans: Perfect for cooking veggies and lean proteins.

- Mason Jars & Glass Containers: Ideal for storing homemade sauces, dressings, and leftovers.
- Grinder for Whole Spices: Freshly ground spices maximize flavor and health benefits.

Understanding Cooking Oils:

Choose oils with anti-inflammatory properties such as:

- Extra Virgin Olive Oil: Rich in monounsaturated fats and antioxidants.
- Avocado Oil:Heart-healthy fats.
- Coconut Oil (in moderation): Contains medium-chain triglycerides.

Plan your grocery trips with anti-inflammatory items in mind:

- Shop the Perimeter: Fresh produce, lean proteins, and nutritious grains are generally found on the perimeter of the supermarket store.
- Buy Seasonal Produce: Seasonal fruits and vegetables are not only fresher but can also be more cheap.

Arrange your kitchen for efficiency and accessibility:

- Store Healthy Snacks at Eye Level: Make it easy to choose nutritious snacks.

- Organize Fridge and Pantry: Keep related things together for easier meal preparation.
- Clear Out Unhealthy Options: Reduce temptation by eliminating processed and sugary foods.

Chapter 2: Meal Planning

Familiarize yourself with the core principles of an anti-inflammatory diet, including the emphasis on whole foods, lean proteins, healthy fats, and a range of fruits and vegetables. Understand which foods have anti-inflammatory characteristics and attempt to include them in your meals.

- Create Balanced Meals: Design your meals to incorporate a balance of macronutrients - carbohydrates, proteins, and fats. Incorporate a range of colorful fruits and vegetables to guarantee a broad spectrum of nutrients and antioxidants.

- Plan for a Week: Start with arranging meals for a week. This helps you keep organized and ensures that you have the appropriate items on hand. in your meal planning Include breakfast, lunch, dinner, and snack.

- Prep Ingredients Ahead: Chop veggies, marinade proteins, and prepare grains ahead of time. Having supplies ready makes it easier to assemble meals during busy days.

- Batch Cooking: Consider batch cooking on weekends. Prepare greater quantities of essentials like grains, meats, and sauces to use throughout the week. This saves time and ensures that you always have a healthful alternative ready.

- Mindful Snacking: Plan for healthy snacks to prevent reaching for processed choices. Options may include: Greek Yogurt with Berries

Vegetable Sticks with Hummus Nuts and Seeds Mix

<u>*Day 1:*</u>

Breakfast:

- Overnight oats with chia seeds, berries, and a scoop of protein powder.

Lunch:

- Quinoa salad with lemon dressing.

Dinner:

- Salmon with roasted veggies (broccoli, Brussels sprouts, sweet potato).

<u>*Day 2:*</u>

Breakfast:

- Scrambled eggs with spinach and whole-wheat bread.

Lunch:

- Chicken quinoa bowl with black beans, corn, chopped veggies, and avocado.

Dinner:

- Lentil soup with whole-wheat bread.

Day 3:

Breakfast:

- Oatmeal with chia seeds, berries, and a drizzle of honey.

Lunch:

- Turkey sandwich on whole-wheat bread with lettuce, tomato, and avocado.

Dinner:

- Vegetarian chili with brown rice and a side salad.

<u>*Day 4:*</u>

Breakfast:

- Smoothie with banana, spinach, protein powder, and unsweetened plant-based milk.

Lunch:

- Chickpea salad sandwich on whole-wheat bread with avocado and sprouts.

Dinner:

- Salmon burgers on whole-wheat buns with sweet potato fries.

<u>*Day 5:*</u>

Breakfast:

- Chia seed pudding with fruit and almond milk.

Lunch:

- Grilled shrimp skewers with a side of quinoa and sautéed spinach.

Dinner:

- Chicken stir-fry with brown rice and mixed vegetables.

Day 6:

Breakfast:

- Spinach and feta omelet.

Lunch:

- Turkey and vegetable wrap on whole-wheat tortilla.

Dinner:

- Vegetarian burgers on whole-wheat buns with sweet potato fries.

Day 7:

Breakfast:

- Scrambled eggs with chopped vegetables and whole-wheat bread.

Lunch:

- Turkey and Avocado Wrap with Whole Grain Tortilla

Dinner:

- Baked cod with roasted broccoli and quinoa.

<u>*Day 8:*</u>

Breakfast:

- Overnight oats with almond milk, chia seeds, mixed fruit

Lunch:

- Chicken Caesar salad with whole-wheat croutons and a light dressing.

Dinner:

- Baked chicken thighs with rosemary, served with rice and roasted Brussels sprouts

---

Day 9:

Breakfast:

- Whole grain bread with smoked salmon, cream cheese, and capers

Lunch:

- Lentil soup with a serving of whole grain crackers

Dinner:

- Grilled veggie and tofu skewers with a side of brown rice

Day 10:

Breakfast:

- Spinach and mushroom frittata
- Whole grain English muffin

Lunch:

- Quinoa salad with black beans, and corn (Avocado-lime dressing)

Dinner:

- Baked cod with lemon-dill

<u>*Day 11:*</u>

Breakfast:

- Smoothie with kale, banana, berries, and a dollop of almond butter
- Whole grain toast with avocado

Lunch:

- Chickpea and vegetable curry with brown rice

Dinner:

- Grilled shrimp with garlic and herb marinade

Day 12:

Breakfast:

- Smoothie with frozen banana, spinach, protein powder, and kefir.

Lunch:

- Quinoa and black bean bowl with roasted veggies(Salsa and avocado topping)

Dinner:

- Stir-fried tofu with bell peppers and broccoli. (Brown rice on the side)

Day 13:

Breakfast:

- Scrambled eggs with sautéed spinach and tomatoes
- Whole grain toast with almond butter

Lunch:

- Quinoa salad with chickpeas, and feta cheese

Dinner:

- Baked salmon with roasted sweet potatoes and steamed broccoli (Quinoa on the side)

<u>*Day 14:*</u>

Breakfast:

- Whole grain toast with smashed avocado and poached egg

Lunch:

- Turkey chili with brown rice and a dollop of Greek yogurt

- Mixed green salad with a balsamic vinaigrette

Dinner:

- Grilled chicken breast with a side of sautéed kale and quinoa

---

Chapter 3: Delicious Anti-Inflammatory Recipes

Breakfast Recipes:

Scrambled Eggs with Spinach

Ingredients:

2 big eggs

1 cup fresh spinach, chopped

1/2 cup cherry tomatoes, halved

Salt and pepper to taste

1 teaspoon olive oil

Preparation:

1. In a bowl, beat the eggs and season with salt and pepper.

2. Warm your olive oil in a pan over medium heat.

3. Add spinach and tomatoes to the skillet, and sauté until spinach wilts.

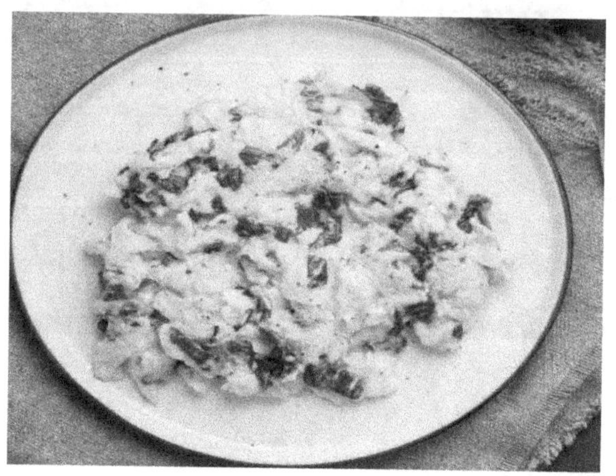

4. Pour beaten eggs over the vegetables and toss until scrambled and heated thoroughly.

5. Serve immediately.

Nutritional Value (approx.):

- Calories: 280, Protein: 18g, Healthy Fats: 20g, Carbohydrates: 10g, Fiber: 3g

Cooking Time: 10 minutes

Serving: 1

Overnight Oats with Almond Milk and Mixed Berries

Ingredients:

1/2 cup rolled oats

1/2 cup unsweetened almond milk

1/2 cup mixed berries (blueberries, strawberries, raspberries)

1 tbsp chia seeds

1 tablespoon chopped walnuts

1 teaspoon honey (optional)

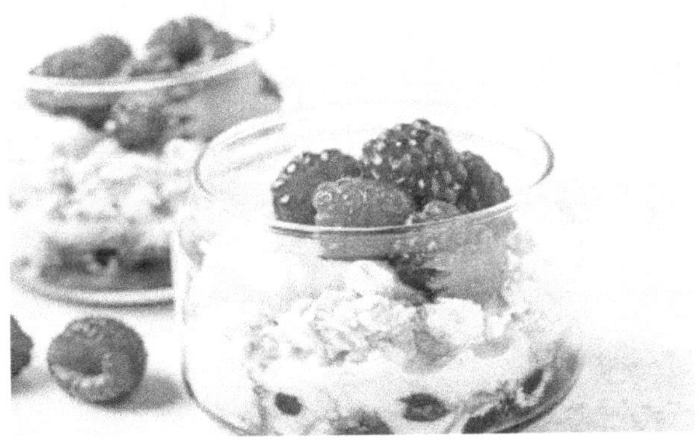

Preparation:

1. In a container, combine oats, almond milk, and chia seeds, and mix thoroughly.
2. Add mixed berries on top and close the container.
3. Refrigerate overnight.
4. In the morning, stir the oats, sprinkle with chopped walnuts, and drizzle with honey if preferred.

Nutritional Value (approx.):

- Calories: 300, Protein: 8g
- Healthy Fats: 15g, Carbohydrates: 35g, Fiber: 9g

Preparation Time: 10 minutes (plus overnight refrigerated)

Serving: 1

Smoothie Bowl with Acai

Ingredients:

1 frozen banana

1/2 cup frozen mixed berries

1 acai berry smoothie pack

1/2 cup almond milk

1 tbsp chia seeds

1/4 cup granola

Sliced fruits for topping (kiwi, strawberries, etc.)

Preparation:

1. In a blender, add frozen banana, mixed berries, acai smoothie pack, and almond milk, and then blend until smooth and pour into a bowl.

2. Top with chia seeds, granola, and sliced fruits and enjoy.

Nutritional Value (approx.):

- Calories: 380, Protein: 7g, Healthy Fats: 15g

- Carbohydrates: 60g, Fiber: 12g

Preparation Time: 5 minutes

Serving: 1

Protein Smoothie

Ingredients:

1 cup unsweetened almond milk

1/2 banana, frozen

1/4 cup mixed berries (fresh or frozen)

1 scoop (25g) protein powder

1 tablespoon chia seeds (optional)

Preparation:

1. Combine all ingredients in a blender and blend until smooth and creamy.
2. Add more liquid if needed to obtain the desired consistency before serving.

Nutritional Value (per serving):

- Calories: 300 , Fat: 8g

- Carbohydrates: 30g, Protein: 25g, Fiber: 3g

Preparation Time: 5 minutes

Serving: 1 person

Berry Chia Seed Pudding

Ingredients:

1/4 cup chia seeds

1 cup unsweetened almond milk

1/4 cup mixed berries (fresh or frozen)

1/4 teaspoon vanilla extract

Optional: 1 tablespoon chopped nuts or seeds, honey/maple syrup to taste

Preparation:

1. In a dish, blend chia seeds, almond milk, berries, and vanilla essence.

2. Stir well and refrigerate for at least 4 hours, or overnight for a thicker consistency.

3. Top with chopped nuts/seeds and drizzle with honey/maple syrup (optional) before serving.

Nutritional Value (per serving):

- Calories: 230 , Fat: 8g
- Carbohydrates: 28g, Protein: 5g
- Fiber: 11g

Preparation Time: 5 minutes

Serving: 1 person

Avocado and Tomato Omelette

Ingredients:

Two big eggs

1/2 avocado, sliced

1/2 cup cherry tomatoes, diced

1 tablespoon olive oil

Salt and pepper to taste

Parsley or chives, chopped (optional) for garnishing

Preparation:

1. In a bowl, beat the eggs and season with salt and pepper.
2. Warm your olive oil in a non-stick pan over medium heat.
3. Pour the beaten eggs into the pan.
4. As the eggs set, add sliced avocado and diced tomatoes to one side.
5. Fold the omelet over the filling and cook until the eggs are fully set.
6. Garnish with fresh herbs if desired. Serve warm.

Nutritional Value:

- Calories: 300, Protein: 14g
- Carbohydrates: 12g , Fat: 24g

Whole Grain Pancakes with Blueberries

Ingredients:

1/2 cup whole wheat flour

1/2 cup almond milk

1 egg

1 teaspoon baking powder

1/2 cup fresh blueberries

Maple syrup for drizzling

Preparation:

1. In a bowl, whisk together whole wheat flour, almond milk, egg, and baking powder until smooth.

2. Heat a non-stick griddle or pan over medium heat.

3. Add 1/4 cup of batter onto the griddle for each pancake.

4. Sprinkle blueberries onto each pancake.

5. Cook until bubbles appear on the surface, then turn and cook the other side until golden brown.

6. Drizzle with maple syrup before serving.

Quantity & Nutritional Value:

- Calories: 250 , Protein: 9g
- Carbohydrates: 40g , Fat: 6g

Cooking Time: 15 minutes

Serving: 2

Whole Grain Toast with Smashed Avocado and Poached Egg

Ingredients:

1 piece whole grain bread

1/2 ripe avocado

1 big egg

Salt and pepper to taste

Red pepper flakes (optional)

Fresh cilantro or chives for garnish (optional)

Preparation:

1. Toast the whole grain bread to your liking.
2. While the bread is toasting, smash the avocado in a bowl and season with salt and pepper.
3. Poach the egg using your preferred method until the yolk is cooked to your desired consistency.
4. Spread the smashed avocado over the toasted bread.
5. Place the poached egg on top.

6. Sprinkle with red pepper flakes for some heat, then garnish with fresh cilantro or chives if preferred.

7. Serve immediately.

Nutritional Value (Approximate):

- Calories: 300-350, Protein: 12g
- Carbohydrates: 20g , Fat: 20g

Cooking Time: 10 minutes

Serving: 1 serving

Spinach and Mushroom Frittata

Ingredients:

3 big eggs

1 cup fresh spinach, chopped

1/2 cup mushrooms, sliced

1/4 cup red bell pepper, diced

1/4 cup feta cheese, crumbled

1 tablespoon olive oil

Salt and pepper to taste

Fresh herbs (such as parsley or thyme), chopped for garnish (optional)

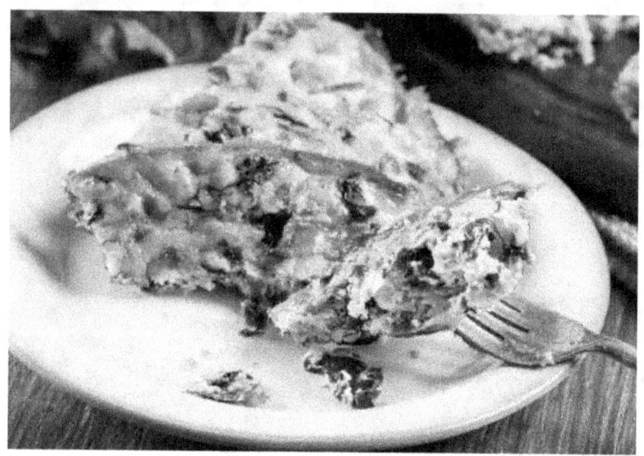

Preparation:

1. Preheat the oven broiler.

2. In a bowl, whisk the eggs and add a little salt and pepper.

3. Warm your olive oil in an oven-safe skillet over medium heat.

4. Add mushrooms and red bell pepper to the skillet, and sauté until tender.

5. Add chopped spinach and simmer until wilted.

6. Pour the whisked eggs into the skillet, ensuring they cover the vegetables equally.

7. Sprinkle crumbled feta cheese on top.

8. Cook on the stovetop for a few minutes until the edges solidify.

9. Transfer the skillet to the oven and broil until the top is golden brown and the middle is firm.

10. Garnish with fresh herbs if desired. Slice and serve warm.

Nutritional Value:

- Calories: 250-300 , Protein: 15g
- Carbohydrates: 8g, Fat: 18g

Cooking Time: 20 minutes

Serving: 2 servings

Whole Grain English Muffin with Almond Butter

Ingredients:

1 whole grain English muffin, toasted

2 tbsp almond butter

1 banana, sliced

Drizzle of honey (optional)

Chia seeds for garnish (optional)

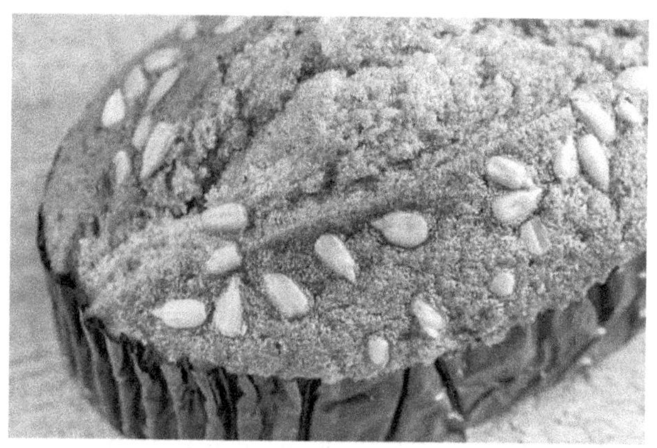

Preparation:

1. Toast the whole-grain English muffin till golden brown.

2. Spread almond butter evenly over each half of the muffin.

3. Set the banana slices on top of the almond butter.

4. Drizzle with honey if preferred and sprinkle with chia seeds for added nutrients.

5. Serve open-faced or as a sandwich.

Nutritional Value (Approximate):

- Calories: 350-400 , Protein: 8g
- Carbohydrates: 40g , Fat: 22g

Cooking Time: 5 minutes

Serving: 1 serving

Lunch Recipes:

Quinoa Salad and Chickpeas

Ingredients:

1 cup cooked quinoa

Half cucumber, diced

one cup of cherry tomatoes, halved

1/2 cup canned chickpeas, drained and rinsed

1/4 cup feta cheese, crumbled

1 tablespoon olive oil

Lemon juice to taste

Salt and pepper to taste

Fresh parsley for garnish (optional)

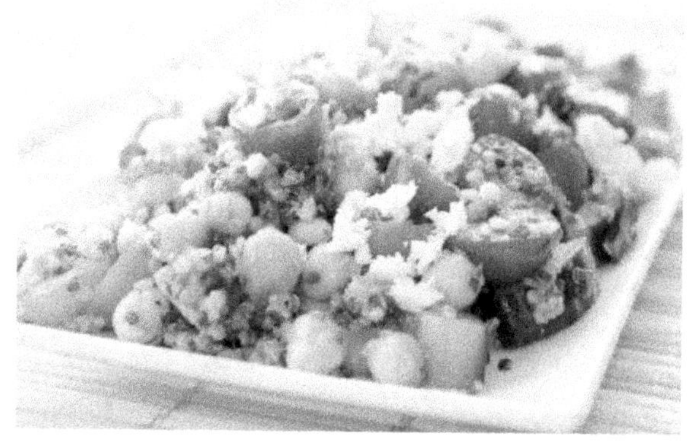

Preparation:

1. In a large bowl, combine cooked quinoa, chopped cucumber, cherry tomatoes, chickpeas, and crumbled feta cheese.

2. Drizzle with olive oil and lemon juice.

3. Season with salt and pepper to taste.

4. Toss the ingredients until fully blended.

5. Garnish with fresh parsley if preferred.

6. Serve at room temperature or chilled.

Nutritional Value:

- Calories: 350 , Protein: 12g
- Carbohydrates: 40g
- Fat: 16g

Preparation Time: 15 minutes

Serving: 2

Turkey and Avocado Wrap

Ingredients:

4 ounces cooked turkey breast, sliced

1 whole grain tortilla

1/2 avocado, sliced

Handful of mixed greens

1 tablespoon Greek yogurt

Lemon juice to taste

Salt and pepper to taste

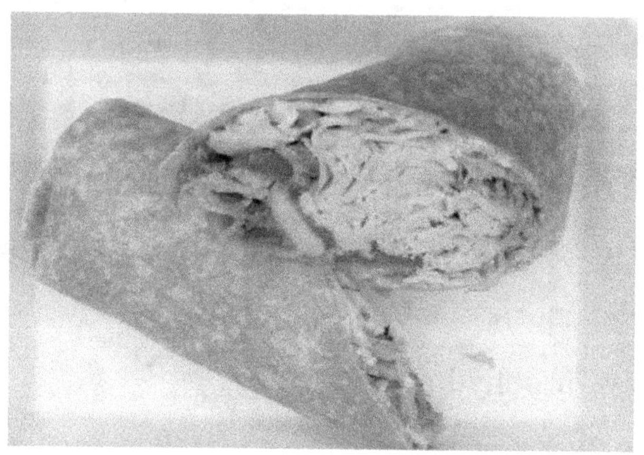

Preparation:

1. Lay the whole-grain tortilla flat.

2. Layer sliced turkey, avocado, and mixed greens on the tortilla.

3. In a small bowl, mix Greek yogurt with lemon juice, salt, and pepper.

4. Drizzle the Greek yogurt mixture over the ingredients.

5. Roll the tortilla into a wrap.

6. Slice in half if desired.

7. Serve immediately.

Nutritional Value:

- Calories: 400, Protein: 25g
- Carbohydrates: 30g, Fat: 20g

Preparation Time: 10 minutes

Serving: 1 serving

Chickpea and Vegetable Stir-Fry with Brown Rice

Ingredients:

1 cup cooked brown rice

1 cup canned chickpeas, drained and rinsed

1 cup broccoli florets

1/2 red bell pepper, sliced

1/2 carrot, julienned

1 tablespoon olive oil

2 teaspoons low-sodium soy sauce

1 teaspoon grated ginger

1 clove garlic, minced

Sesame seeds for garnish (optional)

Green onions for garnish (optional)

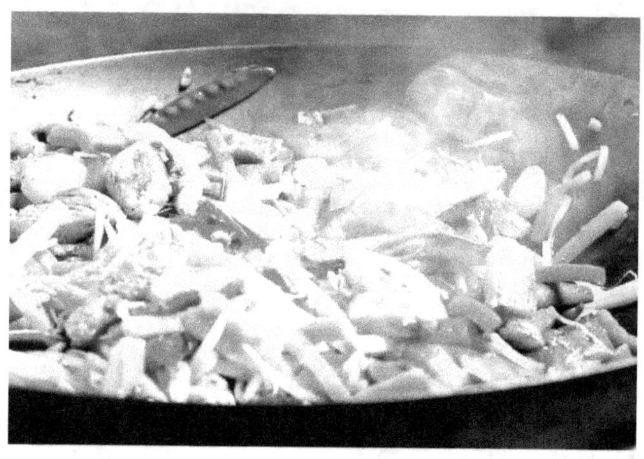

Preparation:

1. Heat your olive oil in a pan over medium heat.

2. Add broccoli, red bell pepper, and julienned carrot. Stir-fry until vegetables are tender-crisp.

3. Add chickpeas to the pan and simmer until heated through.

4. In a small bowl, mix grated ginger, soy sauce, and minced garlic.

5. Pour the sauce over the vegetables and chickpeas. Stir to coat evenly.

6. Serve the stir-fry over a bed of prepared brown rice and then garnish with sesame seeds and green onions if preferred before.

Nutritional Value:

- Calories: 350, Protein: 15g
- Carbohydrates: 50g, Fat: 10g

Preparation Time: 20 minutes

Serving: 2 servings

Tuna Salad Sandwich with Avocado

Ingredients:

2 slices whole-wheat bread

One can (5 oz) of tuna in water, drained and flaked

1/4 avocado, mashed

1 tablespoon chopped celery

1 tablespoon chopped red onion

1 teaspoon lemon juice

Salt and pepper to taste

Preparation:

1. Mash avocado in a bowl. Add flakes tuna, celery, onion, lemon juice, salt, and pepper. Mix well.

2. Spread tuna mixture over one slice of bread and top with the second slice.

Nutritional Value (per serving):

- Calories: 400, Fat: 18g
- Carbohydrates: 35g, Protein: 25g, Fiber: 4g

Cooking Time: 5 minutes

Serving: 1

Lentil Soup

Ingredients:

One cup of dry green lentils, washed

4 cups vegetable broth

1 cup chopped veggies (carrots, celery, onions)

1 clove garlic, minced

1 tablespoon olive oil

1 teaspoon dried thyme

Salt and pepper to taste

1 piece whole-wheat bread

Preparation:

1. Heat your olive oil in a saucepan over medium heat. Add chopped vegetables and simmer for 5 minutes, until softened.

2. Add garlic, lentils, vegetable broth, and thyme. Bring to a boil, then

decrease heat and simmer for 20-25 minutes, or until lentils are cooked.

3. Season with salt and pepper to taste. Eat with a slice of whole-wheat bread.

Nutritional Value (per serving):

- Calories: 350, Fat: 8g
- Carbohydrates: 50g, Protein: 18g, Fiber: 15g

Cooking Time: 30 minutes

Serving: 1

Chicken Caesar Salad with Light Dressing

Ingredients:

Four oz grilled or baked chicken breast, sliced

2 cups mixed greens

1/4 cup cherry tomatoes, halved

1/4 cup grated Parmesan cheese

2 teaspoons light Caesar salad dressing

Croutons (optional, pick whole-wheat or handmade)

Preparation:

1. Arrange mixed greens, tomatoes, and chicken on a platter.
2. Sprinkle with Parmesan cheese and drizzle with light Caesar dressing.
3. Top with croutons (optional) before serving.

Nutritional Value (per serving):

- Calories: 450, Fat: 15g
- Carbohydrates: 20g, Protein: 40g, Fiber: 3g

Preparation Time: 10 minutes (assuming pre-cooked chicken)

Serving: 1 person

Salmon with Roasted Vegetables and Quinoa

Ingredients:

4 ounce salmon filet

1 tablespoon olive oil

1/2 cup chopped broccoli florets

1/2 cup chopped Brussels sprouts

1/4 cup cooked quinoa

Salt and pepper to taste

Lemon wedge (optional)

Preparation:

1. Preheat your oven to 400°F (200°C).
2. Toss broccoli and Brussels sprouts with olive oil, salt, and pepper. Spread on a baking sheet and roast for 15-20 minutes or until tender-crisp.

3. Meanwhile, season the fish with salt and pepper. Heat a pan over medium heat with a drizzle of oil and cook fish for 4-5 minutes per side, or until cooked through.
4. Fluff quinoa with a fork and combine with roasted veggies.
5. Plate fish with quinoa and vegetables. Add a lemon wedge for a fresh touch (optional).

Nutritional Value (per serving):

- Calories: 450, Fat: 20g
- Carbohydrates: 35g, Protein: 30g, Fiber: 5g

Cooking Time: 30 minutes

Serving: 1

Lentil and Vegetable Curry with Brown Rice

Ingredients:

1 cup cooked brown rice

1/2 cup dried lentils, washed and drained

1 cup cauliflower florets

1/2 cup bell peppers, diced

1/2 cup cherry tomatoes, halved

1/4 cup coconut milk

1 tablespoon olive oil

1 teaspoon curry powder

1/2 teaspoon turmeric

Salt and pepper to taste

Fresh cilantro for garnish (optional)

Preparation:

1. In a pot, warm your olive oil over medium heat.

2. Add diced bell peppers, cauliflower florets, and cherry tomatoes. Sauté until slightly softened.

3. Stir in lentils, curry powder, turmeric, salt, and pepper.

4. Pour in coconut milk and carry to a boil.

5. Cover and simmer until the lentils are cooked.

6. Serve the lentil and vegetable curry over a bed of cooked brown rice.

7. Decorate with fresh cilantro if desired before serving.

Nutritional Value per serve:

- Calories: 400
- Protein: 18g, Carbohydrates: 60g, Fat: 10g

Cooking Time: 30 minutes

Serving: 2

Grilled Shrimp Salad with Lemon-Tahini Dressing

Ingredients:

1 cup cooked quinoa

8-10 big shrimp, peeled and deveined

2 cups mixed salad greens

1/2 cucumber, sliced

1/2 cup cherry tomatoes, halved

1/4 cup feta cheese, crumbled

1 tablespoon olive oil

1 tablespoon tahini

Juice of 1 lemon

1 teaspoon honey

Salt and pepper to taste

Preparation:

1. Season shrimp with olive oil, salt, and pepper. Grill till cooked through.

2. In a large bowl, combine cooked quinoa, mixed salad greens, diced cucumber, and cherry tomatoes to

make a salad, and then top the salad with grilled shrimp and crumbled feta cheese.

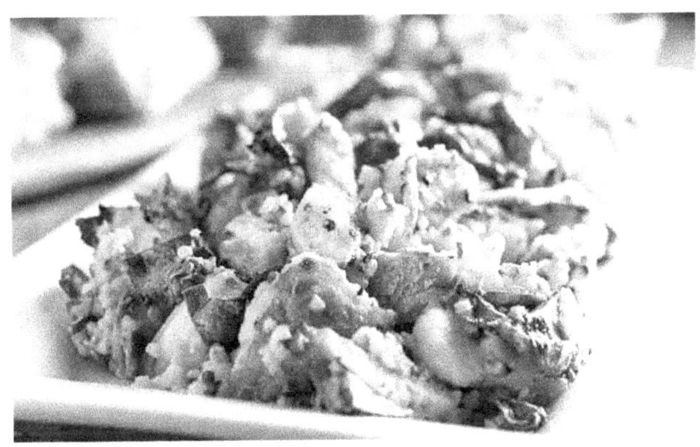

3. In a separate bowl, whisk together tahini, lemon juice, honey, salt, and pepper to make a dressing.
4. Drizzle the dressing over the salad.
5. Toss lightly to mix.
6. Serve immediately.

Nutritional Value per serve:

- Calories: 350 , Protein: 20g
- Carbohydrates: 30g, Fat: 15g

Cooking Time: 20 minutes

Black Bean and Vegetable Chili with Quinoa

Ingredients:

One cup cooked quinoa

Rinsed and drained 1 can (15 oz)of black beans

1 cup bell peppers, chopped (assorted hues)

1 cup zucchini, diced

1 cup corn kernels (fresh or frozen)

One can (14 oz) of sliced tomatoes (low-sodium)

1 cup vegetable broth

1 tablespoon olive oil

1 teaspoon cumin

1 teaspoon chili powder

Salt and pepper to taste

Fresh cilantro for garnish (optional)

Preparation:

1. In a big pot, warm your olive oil over medium heat.

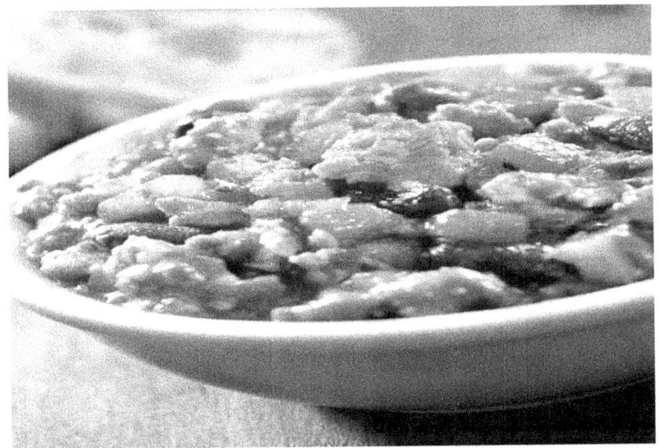

2. Add diced bell peppers and zucchini. Sauté until softened.
3. Stir in cumin, salt, black beans, corn, diced tomatoes, chili powder, and pepper.
4. Pour in veggie broth and bring to a boil.

5. Simmer for 15-20 minutes until the vegetables are soft.

6. Enjoy the chili over a bed of cooked quinoa.

7. Decorate with fresh cilantro if desired.

Nutritional Value per serving:

- Calories: 380 , Protein: 15g
- Carbohydrates: 65g ,Fat: 8g

Cooking Time: 30 minutes

Serving: 2

Salmon and Avocado Bowl with Quinoa

Ingredients:

One cup of cooked quinoa

2 salmon filets

1 avocado, sliced

One cup of cherry tomatoes, halved

1/4 cup red onion, finely diced

1 tablespoon olive oil

Juice of 1 lime

1 teaspoon Dijon mustard

Salt and pepper to taste

Fresh dill for garnish (optional)

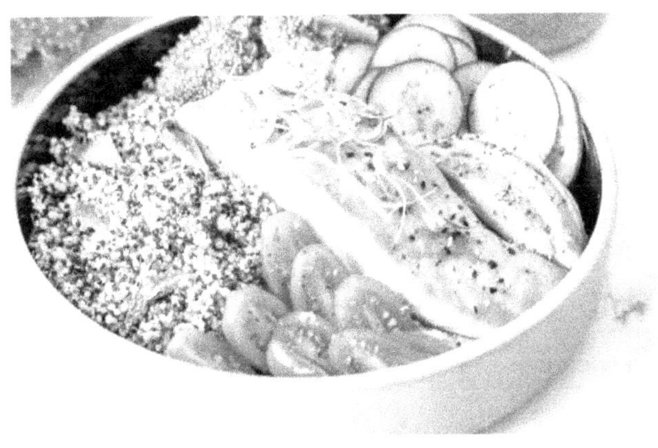

Preparation:

1. Apply salt and pepper on the salmon filets and then grill or bake until cooked through.

2. In a large bowl, add cooked quinoa, sliced avocado, cherry tomatoes, and diced red onion.

3. Whisk together olive oil, lime juice, Dijon mustard, salt, and pepper to make the dressing.

4. Flake the grilled fish and add it to the bowl.

5. Drizzle the dressing over the bowl and stir gently.

6. Garnish with fresh dill if desired.

7. Serve immediately.

Nutritional Value per serving:

- Calories: 420, Protein: 25g
- Carbohydrates: 35g , Fat: 20g

Serving: 2

Dinner Recipes:

Salmon with Roasted Sweet Potatoes and Steamed Broccoli

Ingredients:

2 salmon filets (6 oz each)

2 medium sweet potatoes, peeled and chopped

2 cups broccoli florets

2 tablespoons olive oil

1 teaspoon garlic powder

1 teaspoon dried thyme

Salt and pepper to taste

Lemon wedges for serving

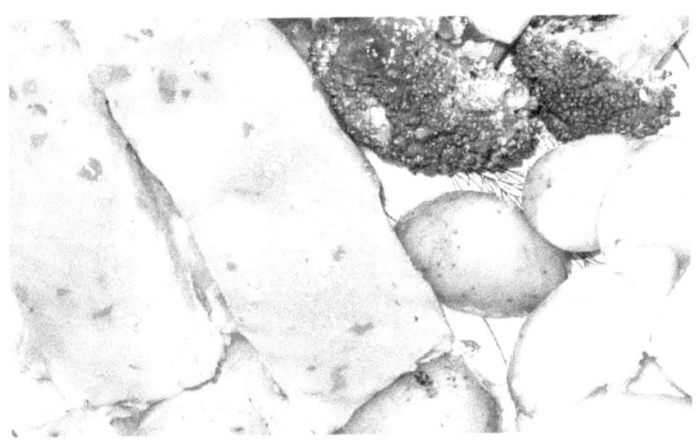

Preparation:

1. Preheat the oven to 400°F (200°C).

2. Place the diced sweet potatoes and broccoli on a baking sheet.

3. Pour slowly with olive oil, and sprinkle with garlic powder, dried thyme, salt, and pepper. Toss to coat evenly.

4. Lay the salmon filets on the same baking sheet.

5. Bake in the preheated oven for 20-25 minutes or until the salmon is cooked through and the vegetables are soft.

6. Serve with lemon wedges for a zesty surge of flavor.

Nutritional Value per serving:

- Calories: 450, Protein: 30g,
- Carbohydrates: 30g, Fat: 22g

Cooking Time: 25 minutes

Serving: 2

Grilled Chicken Breast with Sautéed Kale and Quinoa

Ingredients:

2 boneless, skinless chicken breasts

One bunch of kale stems, removed and the leaves sliced

1 cup cooked quinoa

2 tablespoons olive oil

1 teaspoon lemon zest

1 teaspoon smoked paprika

Salt and pepper to taste

Fresh lemon slices for serving

Preparation:

1. Warm your grill or grill pan over medium-high heat.

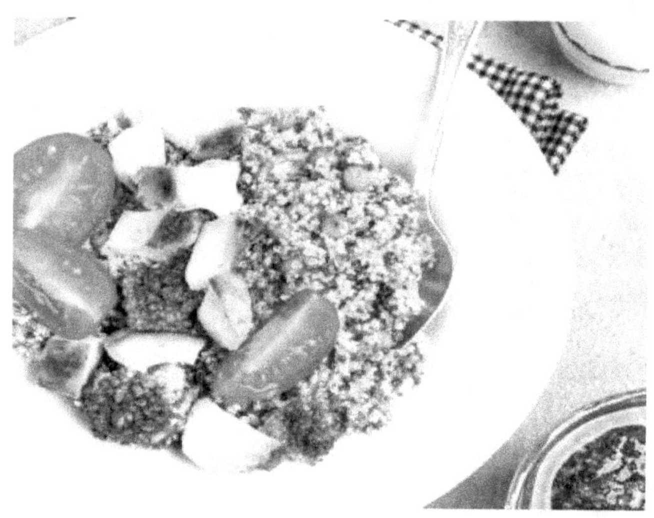

2. Rub chicken breasts with olive oil, lemon zest, smoked paprika, salt, and pepper, and then grill chicken for 6-8 minutes per side or until cooked through.
3. In a pan, warm your olive oil over medium heat. Sauté chopped kale until wilted.
4. Serve grilled chicken over a bed of cooked quinoa with sautéed greens on the side.
5. Garnish with fresh lemon slices.

Nutritional Value per serving:

- Calories: 400, Protein: 35g, Carbohydrates: 25g, Fat: 18g

Cooking Time: 20 minutes

Serving: 2

Stir-fried tofu with Broccoli over Brown Rice

Ingredients:

1 cup firm tofu, cubed

1 cup broccoli florets

1 red bell pepper, thinly sliced

1 yellow bell pepper, thinly sliced

1 green bell pepper, finely sliced

1 cup cooked brown rice

2 tablespoons soy sauce (low-sodium)

1 tablespoon sesame oil

1 teaspoon grated ginger

2 cloves garlic, minced

Sesame seeds for garnish (optional)

Green onions for garnish (optional)

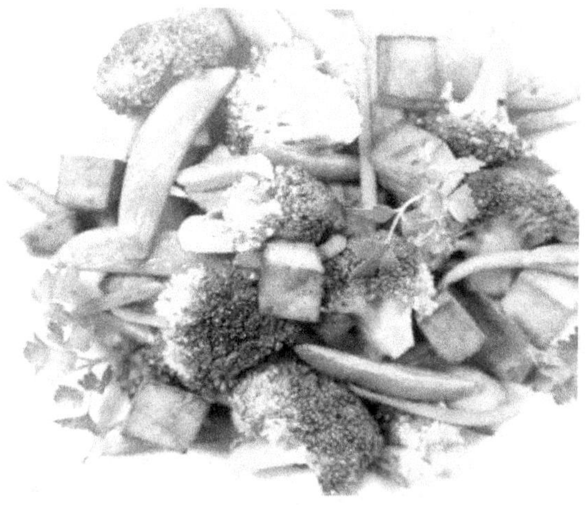

Preparation:

1. In a wok or large pan, warm your sesame oil over medium-high heat.
2. Put cubed tofu and stir-fry until golden brown.
3. Add grated ginger and minced garlic, and stir for 1-2 minutes.
4. Add broccoli, red bell pepper, and yellow bell pepper. Stir-fry until vegetables are tender-crisp.
5. Pour soy sauce over the tofu and vegetables, and mix to incorporate.
6. Serve the stir-fried tofu and vegetables over a bed of prepared brown rice.
7. Decorate with sesame seeds and green onions if preferred.

Nutritional Value per serving:

- Calories: 380 , Protein: 18g

- Carbohydrates: 45g, Fat: 15g

Cooking Time: 15 minutes

Serving: 2 servings

Grilled Turmeric Chicken with Quinoa and Roasted Vegetables

Ingredients:

2 boneless, skinless chicken breasts

1 cup cooked quinoa

1 zucchini, sliced

1 red bell pepper, sliced

1 tablespoon olive oil

1 teaspoon ground turmeric

1 teaspoon smoked paprika

Salt and pepper to taste

Fresh parsley for garnish (optional)

Preparation:

1. Warm your grill or grill pan over medium-high heat.

2. Rub the chicken breasts with olive oil, ground turmeric, smoked paprika, salt, and pepper, and then grill the chicken for 6-8 minutes per side or until cooked through.

3. In a separate skillet, sauté the sliced zucchini and red bell pepper in olive oil until soft.

4. Serve the grilled turmeric chicken over a bed of cooked quinoa with the sautéed vegetables on the side.

5. Decorate with fresh parsley if preferred.

Nutritional Value per serving:

- Calories: 420, Protein: 35g
- Carbohydrates: 35g , Fat: 15g

Cooking Time: 25 minutes

Serving: 2

Bake Salmon and Asparagus with Lemon-Dill Sauce

Ingredients:

2 salmon filets (6 oz each)

1 bunch asparagus, trimmed

2 tablespoons olive oil

1 teaspoon garlic powder

1 teaspoon dried dill

Salt and pepper to taste

Juice of 1 lemon

1 tablespoon Greek yogurt

Fresh dill for garnish (optional)

Preparation:

1. Preheat the oven to 400°F (200°C).
2. Put the salmon filets and trimmed asparagus on a baking sheet.
3. Drizzle with olive oil, and sprinkle with garlic powder, dried dill, salt, and pepper.

4. Bake in the preheated oven for 15-20 minutes or until the salmon is cooked through and the asparagus is soft.

5. In a small dish, mix Greek yogurt with lemon juice to form the sauce.

6. Serve the cooked salmon and asparagus with a drizzle of lemon-dill sauce.

7. Garnish with fresh dill if desired.

Nutritional Value per serving:

- Calories: 380 , Protein: 30g
- Carbohydrates: 15g , Fat: 25g

Cooking Time: 20 minutes

Serving: 2

Mushroom and Spinach Stuffed Bell Peppers with Quinoa

Ingredients:

Two bell peppers, halved and seeds removed

1 cup cooked quinoa

1 cup mushrooms, chopped

2 cups fresh spinach, chopped

1 tablespoon olive oil

1 teaspoon dried oregano

1 teaspoon ground cumin

Salt and pepper to taste

1/4 cup feta cheese, crumbled

Fresh parsley for garnish (optional)

Preparation:

1. Preheat the oven to 375°F (190°C).

2. In a pan, warm your olive oil over medium heat. Sauté mushrooms until tender.

3. Add chopped spinach to the pan and simmer until wilted.

4. In a bowl, mix cooked quinoa with sautéed mushrooms and spinach. Add dried oregano, ground cumin, salt, and pepper.

5. Stir to mix then fill each bell pepper half with the quinoa mixture.

6. Put the stuffed bell peppers on a baking sheet and bake for 20-25 minutes.

7. Sprinkle crumbled feta cheese on top and sprinkle with fresh parsley if preferred before serving.

Nutritional Value per serving:

- Calories: 350 , Protein: 15g
- Carbohydrates: 40g , Fat: 15g

Cooking Time: 30 minutes

Serving: 2

Vegetarian Chili with Brown Rice and a Side Salad

Ingredients:

1 tablespoon olive oil

1 medium onion, chopped

1 green bell pepper, chopped

2 cloves garlic, minced

One (15 oz) can of chopped tomatoes, undrained

One (15 ounces) can of kidney beans, drained and rinsed

Drained and rinsed one (15-ounce) can of black beans

1 cup vegetable broth

1 teaspoon chili powder

1/2 teaspoon cumin

1/4 teaspoon smoked paprika

Salt and pepper to taste

1/2 cup cooked brown rice

Side salad (mixed greens, cucumber, tomato, vinaigrette dressing)

Preparation:

1. Warm your olive oil in a big pot over medium heat. Add onion, and bell pepper, and simmer for 5 minutes, until softened.

2. Add garlic and heat for 30 seconds, until fragrant.

3. Stir in diced tomatoes, kidney beans, black beans, vegetable broth, chili powder, cumin, smoked paprika, salt, and pepper and then carry to a boil, reduce the heat, and simmer for 20 minutes.

4. While chili simmers, prepare your side salad.

5. Serve chili over cooked brown rice and enjoy with a side salad.

Nutritional Value (per serving):

- Calories: 400, Fat: 10g

- Carbohydrates: 50g, Protein: 15g
- Fiber: 15g

Serving: 1

Cooking Time: 40 minutes

Turkey Burgers with Sweet Potato Fries

Ingredients:

1 pound ground turkey

1/4 cup chopped onion

1/4 cup chopped red bell pepper

1 egg, beaten

1/4 cup breadcrumbs

1 tablespoon Worcestershire sauce

1 teaspoon dried thyme

Salt and pepper to taste

1 medium sweet potato, sliced into wedges

Olive oil spray

2 whole-wheat hamburger buns

Toppings of your choosing (lettuce, tomato, avocado, etc.)

Preparation:

1. Preheat the oven to 400°F (200°C).
2. In a large bowl, combine ground turkey, onion, bell pepper, egg, breadcrumbs, Worcestershire sauce, thyme, salt, and pepper. Mix well.
3. Form the ingredients into two burger patties.

4. Place sweet potato wedges on a baking sheet, drizzle with olive oil, and season with salt and pepper. Roast for 20-25 minutes, or until tender-crisp.

5. Warm your grill pan or skillet over medium heat. Cook burgers for 4-5 minutes per side, or until cooked through.

6. Toast whole-wheat buns if desired.

7. Assemble burgers on buns with your choice of toppings. Enjoy with sweet potato fries.

Nutritional Value (per serving):

- Calories: 500 , Fat: 20g
- Carbohydrates: 40g, Protein: 40g
  Fiber: 5g

Serving: 1

Vegetarian Chickpea and Spinach Curry with Brown Rice

Ingredients:

1 cup cooked brown rice

Rinsed and drained one can (15 oz) of chickpeas

2 cups fresh spinach

1 big tomato, chopped

1 onion, finely chopped

2 cloves garlic, minced

1 tablespoon olive oil

1 teaspoon ground cumin

1 teaspoon ground coriander

1/2 teaspoon turmeric

1/2 teaspoon paprika

Salt and pepper to taste

Fresh cilantro for garnish (optional)

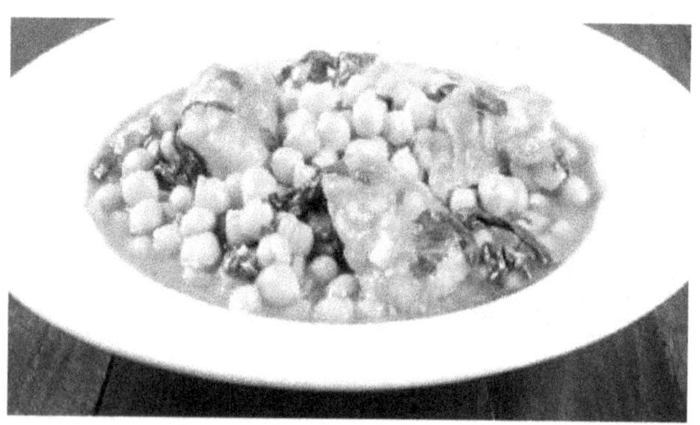

Preparation:

1. In a pan, warm your olive oil over medium heat. Put chopped onions and sauté until transparent.

2. Put minced garlic and sauté for an additional minute.

3. Stir in ground cumin, ground coriander, turmeric, paprika, salt, and pepper.

4. Add diced tomatoes and simmer until softened.

5. Add chickpeas and fresh spinach. Stir until the spinach wilts.

6. Serve the chickpea and spinach curry over a bed of cooked brown rice.

7. Decorate with fresh cilantro if desired.

Nutritional Value per serving:

- Calories: 380 , Protein: 15g
- Carbohydrates: 60g , Fat: 10g

Cooking Time: 25 minutes

Serving: 2

Lemon Herb Grilled Shrimp with Quinoa and Asparagus

Ingredients:

1 cup cooked quinoa

8-10 large shrimp, peeled and deveined

1 bunch asparagus, trimmed

2 tablespoons olive oil

Juice of 1 lemon

1 teaspoon dried thyme

1 teaspoon dried rosemary

Salt and pepper to taste

Lemon wedges for serving

Preparation:

1. Warm your grill or grill pan over medium-high heat.

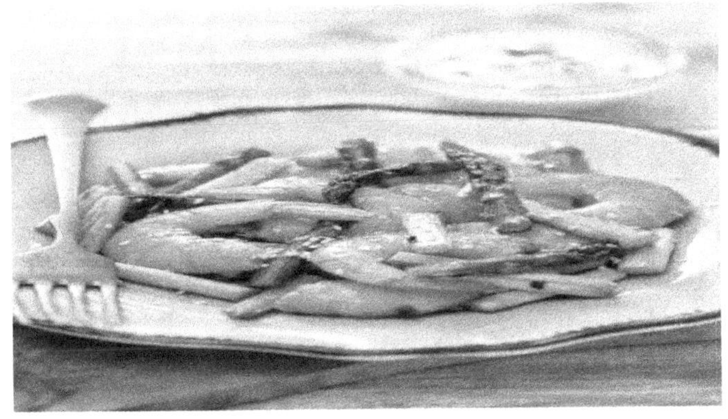

2. In a bowl, combine shrimp and trimmed asparagus with olive oil, lemon juice, dried thyme, dried rosemary, salt, and pepper.

3. Grill the shrimp for 2-3 minutes per side or until opaque and the asparagus until soft.

4. Serve the grilled shrimp and asparagus over a bed of prepared quinoa.

5. Decorate with lemon wedges for an added punch of flavor.

Nutritional Value per serving:

- Calories: 400, Protein: 25g
- Carbohydrates: 30g, Fat: 20g

Cooking Time: 15 minutes

Serving: 2

Poultry Recipes:

Orange Glazed Chicken with Roasted Brussels Sprouts

Ingredients:

Two boneless, skinless chicken thighs

1 cup quinoa, washed

1 pound Brussels sprouts, halved

2 tablespoons olive oil

Zest and juice of 1 orange

1 tablespoon honey

1 teaspoon ground turmeric

Salt and pepper to taste

Fresh thyme for garnish (optional)

Preparation:

1. Preheat the oven to 400°F (200°C).
2. Season chicken thighs with olive oil, orange zest, honey, ground turmeric, salt, and pepper.
3. Place the chicken on a baking sheet along with halved Brussels sprouts.
4. Roast in the oven for 25-30 minutes or until the chicken is cooked through and Brussels sprouts are crunchy.
5. In a saucepan, prepare quinoa according to package instructions.
6. Serve the orange-glazed chicken over a bed of cooked quinoa with roasted Brussels sprouts on the side.
7. Garnish with fresh thyme if preferred.

Nutritional Value preserving:

- Calories: 420, Protein: 25g
- Carbohydrates: 40g, Fat: 18g

Cooking Time: 35 minutes

Serving: 2

Baked Lemon Herb Turkey Meatballs with Zucchini Noodles

Ingredients:

1 pound ground turkey

2 zucchinis, spiralized into noodles

1/4 cup almond flour

1 egg

2 tablespoons olive oil

Juice of 1 lemon

1 teaspoon dried thyme

1 teaspoon dried rosemary

Salt and pepper to taste

Fresh parsley for garnish (optional)

Preparation:

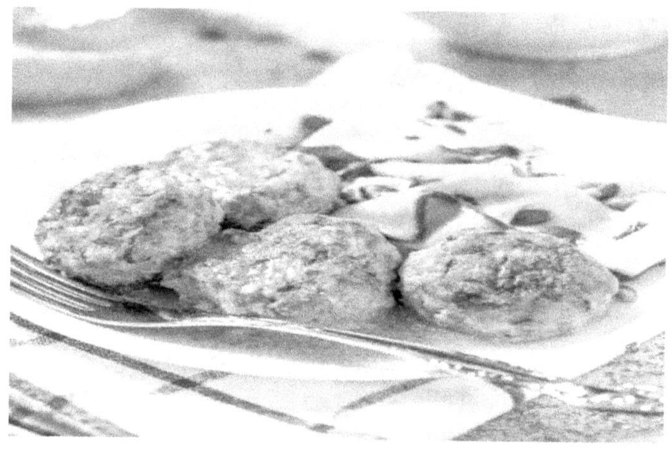

1. Preheat the oven to 375°F (190°C).

2. In a bowl, combine ground turkey, almond flour, egg, olive oil, lemon juice, dried thyme, dried rosemary, salt, and pepper. Mix well.

3. Form the mixture into meatballs, lay them on a baking pan and then bake in the preheated oven for 20-25 minutes or until the meatballs are cooked through.

4. In a pan, sauté zucchini noodles with olive oil until just soft.

5. Serve the baked lemon herb turkey meatballs over a bed of zucchini noodles.

6. Garnish with fresh parsley if preferred.

Nutritional Value:

- Calories: 380 , Protein: 30g
- Carbohydrates: 15g, Fat: 22g

Cooking Time: 30 minutes

Serving: 2

Curry Chicken and Vegetable Skewers

Ingredients:

Two boneless, skinless chicken breasts, cut into cubes

1 cup cooked quinoa

1 bell pepper, cut into pieces

1 zucchini, sliced

1 red onion, cut into bits

2 tablespoons olive oil

1 tablespoon curry powder

1 teaspoon ground cumin

1 teaspoon paprika

Salt and pepper to taste

Fresh cilantro for garnish (optional)

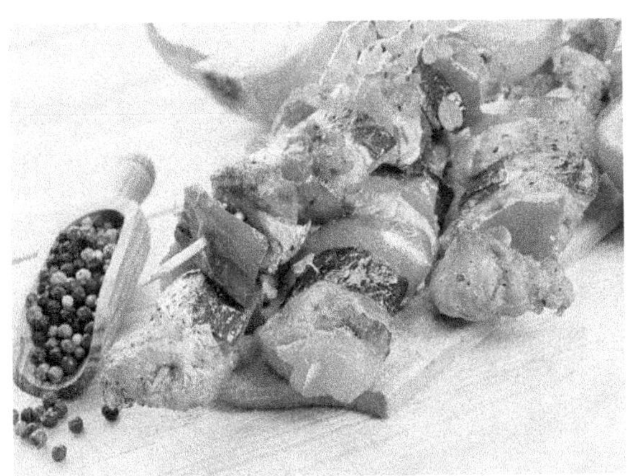

Preparation:

1. In a bowl, blend olive oil, curry powder, ground cumin, paprika, salt, and pepper.

2. Thread chicken cubes, bell pepper chunks, zucchini slices, and red onion chunks onto skewers.

3. Brush the skewers with the curry-spiced oil mixture.

4. Grill the skewers on medium-high heat for 10-15 minutes, flipping regularly, until the chicken is cooked through.

5. Serve the curry chicken and veggie skewers over a bed of cooked quinoa.

6. Decorate with fresh cilantro if desired.

Nutritional Value:

- Calories: 400, Protein: 30g
- Carbohydrates: 40g, Fat: 15g

Cooking Time: 20 minutes

Serving: 2

Herb-Roasted Chicken and Steamed Vegetables

Ingredients:

Two bone-in, skin-on chicken breasts

1 cup quinoa, washed

2 cups mixed vegetables (such as broccoli, carrots, and bell peppers)

2 tablespoons olive oil

1 teaspoon dried thyme

1 teaspoon dried rosemary

1 teaspoon garlic powder

Salt and pepper to taste

Fresh parsley for garnish (optional)

Preparation:

1. Preheat the oven to 400°F (200°C).

2. Rub chicken breasts with olive oil, dried thyme, dried rosemary, garlic powder, salt, and pepper.

3. Place the chicken on a baking sheet and roast for 25-30 minutes or until the internal temperature reaches 165°F (74°C).

4. In a saucepan, prepare quinoa according to package instructions.

5. Steam mixed vegetables till tender-crisp.

6. Serve the herb-roasted chicken over a bed of cooked quinoa with steamed veggies on the side.

7. Decorate with fresh parsley if preferred.

Nutritional Value:

- Calories: 450, Protein: 30g

- Carbohydrates: 40g
- Fat: 18g

Cooking Time: 35 minutes

Serving: 2

Turkey and Vegetable Stir-Fry with Brown Rice

Ingredients:

1 cup cooked brown rice

half pound of ground turkey

1 cup broccoli florets

1/2 red bell pepper, sliced

1/2 yellow bell pepper, sliced

2 teaspoons low-sodium soy sauce

1 tablespoon olive oil

1 teaspoon grated ginger

1 clove garlic, minced

Sesame seeds for garnish (optional)

Green onions for garnish (optional)

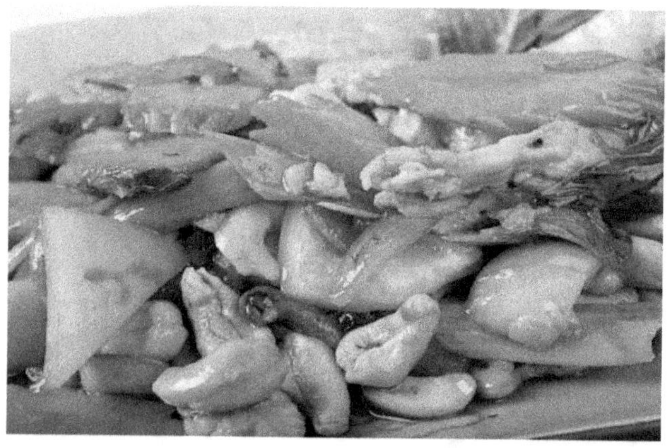

Preparation:

1. In a big pan or wok, warm your olive
   oil over medium-high heat.

2. Add ground turkey and heat until
   browned.

3. Add broccoli, red bell pepper, and yellow bell pepper to the pan. Stir-fry until vegetables are tender-crisp.

4. In a small bowl, mix soy sauce, grated ginger, and minced garlic.

5. Pour the sauce over the turkey and vegetables. Stir to coat evenly.

6. Serve the turkey and veggie stir-fry over a bed of cooked brown rice.

7. Garnish with sesame seeds and green onions if preferred.

Nutritional Value per serving:

- Calories: 380, Protein: 25g
- Carbohydrates: 40g, Fat: 15g

Cooking Time: 20 minutes

Serving: 2

Chicken Fajitas with Whole-Wheat Tortillas

Ingredients:

1 tablespoon olive oil

One pound skinless, boneless chicken breasts, sliced thin

1 bell pepper (any color), cut

1/2 onion, sliced

1 teaspoon chili powder

1/2 teaspoon cumin

1/4 teaspoon smoked paprika

Salt and pepper to taste

2 whole-wheat tortillas Guacamole (for serving)

Toppings of your choosing (shredded lettuce, chopped tomatoes, diced avocado, salsa, etc.)

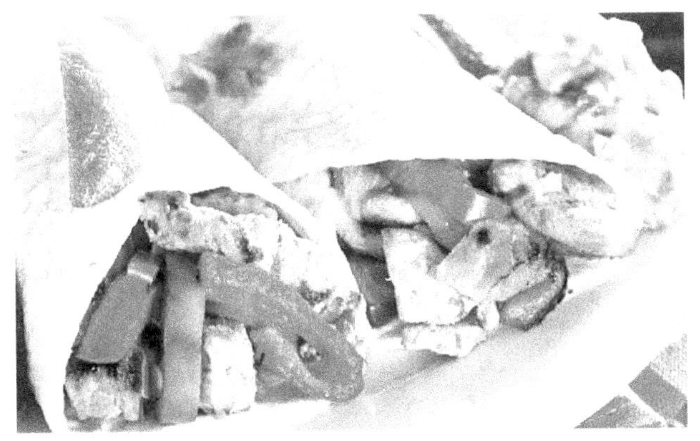

Preparation:

1. Heat olive oil in a large skillet or grill pan over medium-high heat.

2. Add chicken, bell pepper, and onion. Cook for 5-7 minutes, stirring periodically, until chicken is cooked through and veggies are softened.

3. Sprinkle chili powder, cumin, smoked paprika, salt, and pepper over the chicken and vegetables. Stir to coat.

4. Warm whole-wheat tortillas according to package instructions.

5. Fill tortillas with chicken and veggie mixture. Top with guacamole and your choice of toppings.

Nutritional Value:

- Calories: 400 , Fat: 15g
- Carbohydrates: 35g, Protein: 40g
- Fiber: 2g

Cooking Time: 15 minutes

Serving: 1

Seafood Recipes:

Garlic Herb Baked Cod and Roasted Vegetables

Ingredients:

2 fish filets (6 oz each)

1 cup quinoa, washed

1 cup cherry tomatoes, halved

1 zucchini, sliced

 2 tablespoons olive oil

2 cloves garlic, minced

1 teaspoon dried thyme

1 teaspoon dried rosemary

Salt and pepper to taste

Fresh parsley for garnish (optional)

Preparation:

1. Preheat the oven to 400°F (200°C).

2. In a bowl, mix olive oil, minced garlic, dried thyme, dried rosemary, salt, and pepper.

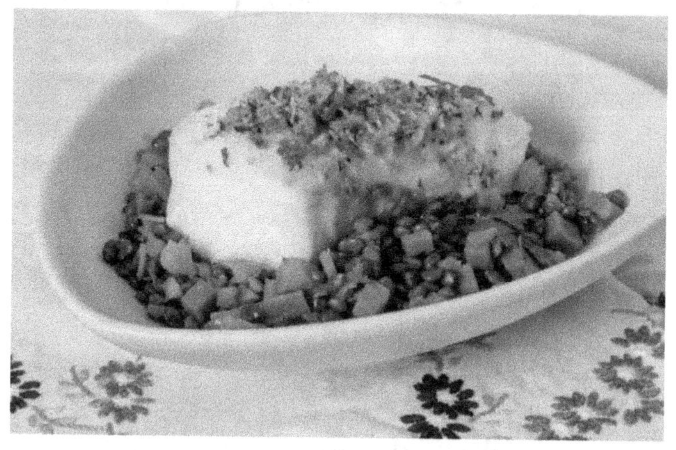

3. Place cod filets on a baking sheet. Brush the filets with the garlic herb mixture.

4. Surround the cod with half cherry tomatoes and sliced zucchini then bake in the preheated oven for 15-20 minutes or until the fish is cooked through and flakes easily.

5. In a saucepan, prepare quinoa according to package instructions.

6. Serve the garlic herb-baked cod over a bed of cooked quinoa with roasted veggies on the side.

7. Decorate with fresh parsley if preferred.

Nutritional Value:

- Calories: 380, Protein: 30g
- Carbohydrates: 40g, Fat: 15g

Cooking Time: 25 minutes

Serving: 2

Spicy Shrimp Stir-Fry with Brown Rice

Ingredients:

1 cup cooked brown rice

8-10 big shrimp, peeled and deveined

1 cup broccoli florets

1/2 bell pepper, cut

1/2 cup snap peas

2 tablespoons soy sauce (low-sodium)

1 tablespoon olive oil

1 teaspoon Sriracha sauce (modify to taste)

1 teaspoon grated ginger

2 cloves garlic, minced

Sesame seeds for garnish (optional)

Green onions for garnish (optional)

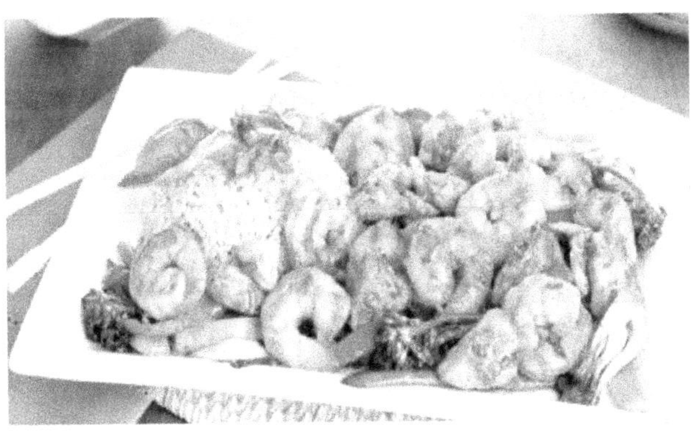

Preparation:

1. In a wok or large pan, warm your olive oil over medium-high heat.

2. Add shrimp and stir-fry until pink and opaque. Remove shrimp from the pan.

3. In the same pan, add broccoli, bell pepper, and snap peas. Stir-fry until vegetables are tender-crisp.

4. Add back the cooked shrimp.

5. In a small bowl, mix soy sauce, Sriracha sauce, grated ginger, and minced garlic.

6. Pour the sauce over the shrimp and vegetables. Stir to mix.

7. Serve the spicy shrimp stir-fry over a bed of cooked brown rice.

8. Decorate with sesame seeds and green onions if preferred.

Nutritional Value:

- Calories: 350, Protein: 20g
- Carbohydrates: 35g, Fat: 15g

Cooking Time: 20 minutes

Serving: 2

Shrimp Scampi with Zucchini Noodles

Ingredients:

1 tablespoon olive oil

1 clove garlic, minced

1/2 cup chopped red onion

1/4 cup dry white wine (optional)

1 cup cherry tomatoes, halved

1/2 teaspoon dried oregano

1/4 teaspoon red pepper flakes (optional)

12 ounces raw shrimp, peeled and deveined

1 (12 oz) package spiralized zucchini (or zucchini noodles)

Salt and pepper to taste

Chopped fresh parsley (optional, for garnish)

Preparation:

1. Warm your olive oil in a large skillet over medium heat. Add garlic and red onion. Cook for 3-4 minutes, until softened.

2. Add white wine (if using) and simmer for 1 minute, scraping up any browned bits from the bottom of the pan.

3. Stir in cherry tomatoes, oregano, and red pepper flakes (if using). Bring to a simmer and cook for 5 minutes, until tomatoes soften slightly.

4. Add shrimp and heat for 3-4 minutes, or until pink and cooked through. Season with salt and pepper.

5. Meanwhile, cook zucchini noodles according to package instructions or until tender-crisp. Drain and set aside.

6. Serve shrimp scampi over zucchini noodles and sprinkle with chopped parsley (optional).

Nutritional Value (per serving):

- Calories: 350, Fat: 10g
- Carbohydrates: 25g, Protein: 30g
- Fiber: 3g

Cooking Time: 15 minutes

Serving: 1

Miso-glazed halibut and Stir-Fried Bok Choy

Ingredients:

2 halibut filets (approximately 6 oz each)

1 cup quinoa, washed

1 bunch baby bok choy, cut

2 tablespoons miso paste

1 tablespoon soy sauce (low-sodium)

1 tablespoon rice vinegar

1 tablespoon honey

1 teaspoon sesame oil

2 cloves garlic, minced

1 teaspoon grated ginger

Sesame seeds for garnish (optional)

Green onions for garnish (optional)

Preparation:

1. In a bowl, mix miso paste, soy sauce, rice vinegar, honey, sesame oil, minced garlic, and grated ginger.

2. Brush the halibut filets with the miso glaze. Warm your grill or grill pan over medium-high heat. Grill the halibut for 4-5 minutes per side or until it flakes easily.

3. In a saucepan, prepare quinoa according to package instructions.

4. In a separate skillet, stir-fry chopped bok choy until barely wilted.

5. Serve the miso-glazed halibut over a bed of cooked quinoa with stir-fried bok cabbage on the side.

6. Decorate with sesame seeds and green onions if preferred.

Nutritional Value:

- Calories: 420 , Protein: 30g
- Carbohydrates: 40g, Fat: 15g

Cooking Time: 25 minutes

Serving: 2

Coconut Lime Shrimp Skewers with Turmeric Cauliflower Rice

Ingredients:

1 pound large shrimp, peeled and deveined

1 cauliflower, grated (for cauliflower rice)

1 can (14 oz) coconut milk

Juice of 2 limes

1 tablespoon olive oil

1 teaspoon ground turmeric

1 teaspoon curry powder

Salt and pepper to taste

Fresh cilantro for garnish (optional)

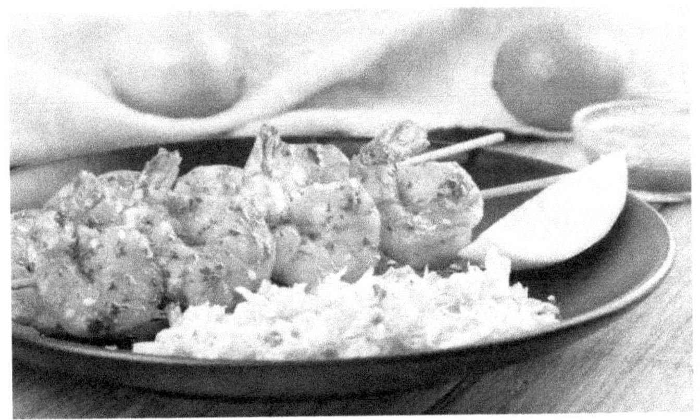

Preparation:

1. In a bowl, marinate shrimp with coconut milk, lime juice, olive oil, ground turmeric, curry powder, salt, and pepper.

2. Thread the marinated shrimp on skewers.

3. Warm your grill or grill pan over medium-high heat. Grill the shrimp

skewers for 2-3 minutes per side or until opaque.

4. In a pan, sauté grated cauliflower with a touch of olive oil until it resembles rice. Season with salt and pepper.

5. Serve the coconut lime shrimp skewers over turmeric cauliflower rice.

6. Decorate with fresh cilantro if desired.

Nutritional Value:

- Calories: 380 , Protein: 25g
- Carbohydrates: 15g, Fat: 20g

Cooking Time: 20 minutes

Serving: 2

Greek-Style Grilled Octopus Salad with Quinoa

Ingredients:

2 octopus tentacles

1 cup quinoa, washed

1 cucumber, diced

1 cup cherry tomatoes, halved

1/4 cup Kalamata olives, sliced

2 tablespoons olive oil

Juice of 1 lemon

1 teaspoon dried oregano

Salt and pepper to taste

Fresh parsley for garnish (optional)

Preparation:

1. Warm your grill or grill pan over medium-high heat. Grill the octopus tentacles for 3-4 minutes per side or until cooked through.

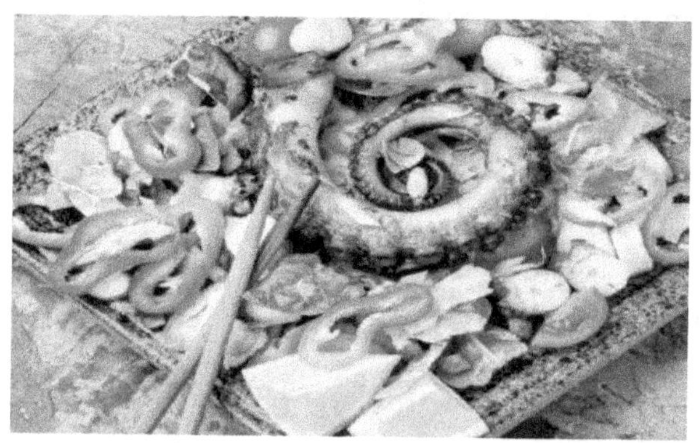

2. In a saucepan, prepare quinoa according to package instructions.

3. Slice grilled octopus tentacles into bite-sized pieces.

4. In a bowl, add cooked quinoa, chopped cucumber, cherry tomatoes, sliced Kalamata olives, and octopus pieces.

5. Drizzle the salad with olive oil, lemon juice, dried oregano, salt, and pepper. Toss to blend.

6. Serve the Greek-style grilled octopus salad over a bed of quinoa.

7. Decorate with fresh parsley if preferred.

Nutritional Value per serving:

- Calories: 400, Protein: 25g
- Carbohydrates: 40g, Fat: 18g

Cooking Time: 25 minutes

Serving: 2

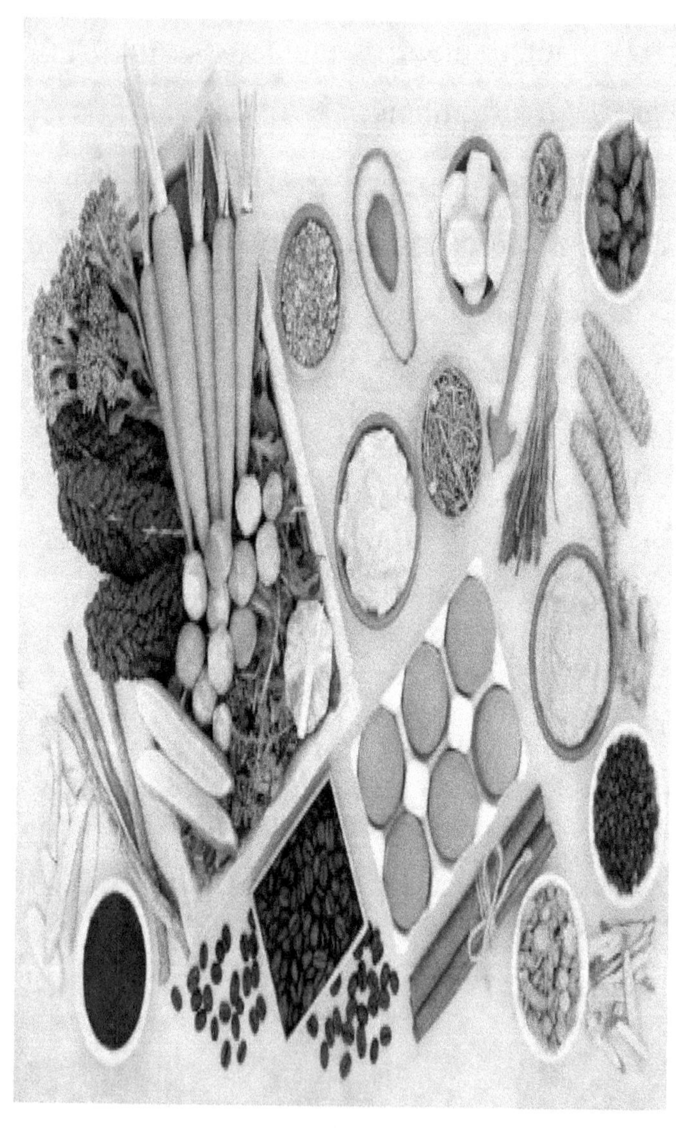

Chapter 5: Special Diets and Dietary Modifications

Plant-based Protein Sources Recipes:

Tofu Scramble with Vegetables

Ingredients:

One block (14 oz) of firm tofu, drained and pressed

1 tablespoon olive oil

Half onion chopped

half bell pepper (any color), chopped

1/4 cup chopped mushrooms

1/4 teaspoon turmeric powder

1/4 teaspoon smoked paprika

Salt and pepper to taste

Chopped fresh herbs (optional, for garnish)

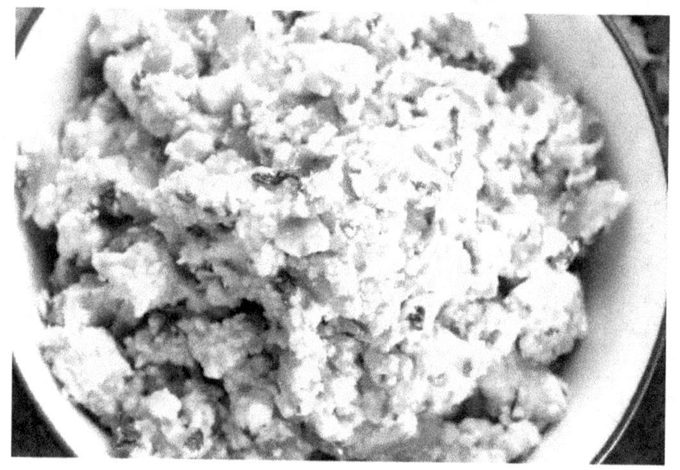

Preparation:

1. Crumble tofu with your hands or a fork.

2. Warm your olive oil in a pan over medium heat and then add onion, bell pepper, and mushrooms. Cook for 5 minutes, until softened.

3. Add crumbled tofu, turmeric, smoked paprika, salt, and pepper. Cook for another 5 minutes, stirring periodically, until cooked thoroughly.

4. Serve tofu scramble warm with your choice of toppings like avocado slices, salsa, or chopped fresh herbs.

Nutritional Value (per serving):

- Calories: 300, Fat: 12g
- Carbohydrates: 20g, Protein: 20g, Fiber: 2g

Cooking Time: 15 minutes

Serving: 1

Black Bean Burgers with Sweet Potato Fries

Ingredients:

For the black bean burgers:

1 (15 ounce) can black beans, washed and drained

1/2 cup cooked brown rice

1/4 cup chopped red onion

1/4 cup chopped cilantro

1 tablespoon breadcrumbs

1 teaspoon chili powder

1/2 teaspoon cumin

Salt and pepper to taste

For the sweet potato fries:

1 medium sweet potato, sliced into wedges

1 tablespoon olive oil

Salt and pepper to taste

Preparation:

1. Make the black bean burgers: In a food processor, pulse black beans, brown rice, red onion, cilantro, breadcrumbs, chili powder, cumin, salt, and pepper until mixed but still slightly chunky.
2. Form the ingredients into two burger patties.
3. Warm your grill pan or skillet over medium heat. Cook the burgers for 4-5 minutes per side, or until heated through.

4. Make the sweet potato fries: Preheat the oven to 400°F (200°C) and then toss sweet potato wedges with olive oil, salt, and pepper. Spread on a baking sheet and bake for 20-25 minutes, or until tender-crisp.

5. Serve black bean burgers on buns with your favorite toppings and eat with sweet potato fries.

Nutritional Value (per serving):

- Calories: 500, Fat: 15g
- Carbohydrates: 50g, Protein: 20g, Fiber: 10g

Cooking Time: 40 minutes

Serving: 1

Lentil and Mushroom Stuffed Bell Peppers with Wild Rice

Ingredients:

1 cup wild rice, cooked

One cup of brown lentils, cooked

Two bell peppers, halved and seeds removed

1 cup mushrooms, finely chopped

1 onion, finely chopped

Two cloves garlic, minced

1 tablespoon olive oil

1 teaspoon dried thyme

1 teaspoon smoked paprika

Salt and pepper to taste

Tomato sauce for topping

Preparation:

1. Preheat the oven to 375°F (190°C).

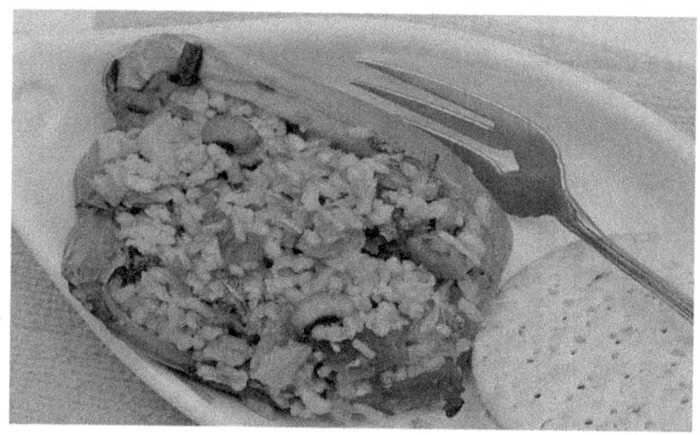

2. In a pan, warm your olive oil over medium heat. Sauté onions and garlic until transparent.

3. Add chopped mushrooms to the pan and simmer until softened.

4. In a bowl, mix cooked wild rice, cooked lentils, sautéed mushrooms, dried thyme, smoked paprika, salt, and pepper.

5. Stuff each bell pepper half with the lentil and mushroom mixture.

6. Place the stuffed bell peppers in a baking tray, sprinkle them with tomato sauce and then bake in the preheated oven for 20-25 minutes or until the peppers are cooked.

Nutritional Value per serving:

- Calories: 380, Protein: 20g
- Carbohydrates: 60g, Fat: 8g

Cooking Time: 30 minutes

Serving: 2

Quinoa and Black Bean Stuffed Zucchini Boats

Ingredients:

2 medium-sized zucchini

1 cup quinoa, cooked

Rinsed and drained one can (15 oz) of black beans

1 cup corn kernels

One cup of cherry tomatoes, halved

1/2 red onion, coarsely chopped

Two tablespoons of olive oil

Juice of 1 lime

1 teaspoon cumin

1 teaspoon chili powder

Salt and pepper to taste

Fresh cilantro for garnish (optional)

Preparation:

1. Preheat the oven to 375°F (190°C).

2. Cut zucchini in half lengthwise and scoop out the seeds to create a hollow "boat."

3. In a bowl, mix cooked quinoa, black beans, corn, cherry tomatoes, red onion, olive oil, lime juice, cumin, chili powder, salt, and pepper.

4. Fill each zucchini boat with the quinoa and black bean mixture and then place the stuffed zucchini boats in your baking dish and bake in the preheated oven for 20-25 minutes or until the zucchini is soft.

5. Decorate with fresh cilantro if desired.

Nutritional Value per serving:

- Calories: 350, Protein: 15g
- Carbohydrates: 60g, Fat: 8g

Cooking Time: 30 minutes

Serving: 2

Quinoa Black Bean Buddha Bowl with Avocado Lime Dressing

Ingredients:

1 cup quinoa, washed

Rinsed and drained one can (15 oz) of black beans

2 cups mixed greens (spinach, kale, arugula)

1 avocado, sliced

1 cup cherry tomatoes, halved

1/4 cup red onion, finely chopped

2 tablespoons olive oil

Juice of 1 lime

1 teaspoon ground cumin

1 teaspoon chili powder

Salt and pepper to taste

Fresh cilantro for garnish (optional)

Preparation:

1. In a saucepan, prepare quinoa according to package instructions.
2. In a bowl, mix black beans with ground cumin, chili powder, salt, and pepper.
3. In a large serving bowl, arrange cooked quinoa, seasoned black beans,

mixed greens, sliced avocado, split cherry tomatoes, and chopped red onion.

4. In a small bowl, whisk together olive oil and lime juice to produce the dressing.

5. Drizzle the avocado lime dressing over the Buddha bowl.

6. Garnish with fresh cilantro if desired.

Nutritional Value per serving:

- Calories: 420, Protein: 15g
- Carbohydrates: 55g, Fat: 20g

Cooking Time: 20 minutes

Serving: 2

Chickpea and Vegetable Stew with Quinoa

Ingredients:

1 cup quinoa, rinsed

Rinsed and drained one can (15 oz) of chickpeas

Two carrots, peeled and chopped

1 zucchini, diced

1 bell pepper, diced

1 onion, finely chopped

2 cloves garlic, minced

1 can (14 oz) crushed tomatoes

4 cups vegetable broth

1 teaspoon ground cumin

1 teaspoon smoked paprika

Salt and pepper to taste

Fresh cilantro for garnish (optional)

Preparation:

1. In a large pot, sauté your minced garlic and chopped onion until softened.

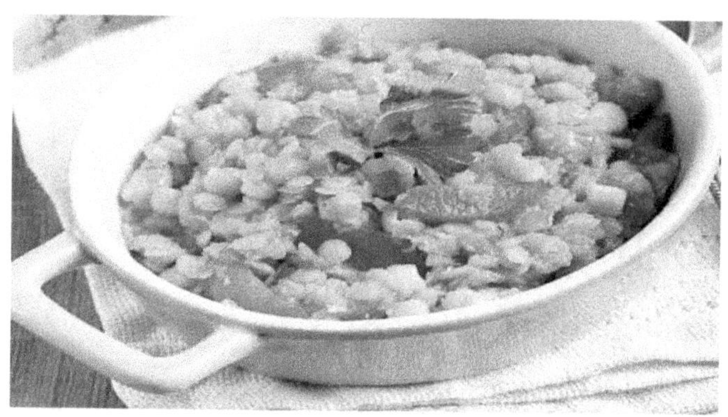

2. Put diced carrots, zucchini, and bell pepper. Cook until vegetables start to soften.

3. Stir in ground cumin, smoked paprika, salt, and pepper.

4. Add chickpeas, smashed tomatoes, and vegetable broth, and then bring to a simmer and let it cook for 20-25 minutes.

5. In a separate saucepan, cook quinoa according to the instructions written in the package.

6. Serve the chickpea and vegetable stew over a bed of cooked quinoa.

7. Garnish with fresh cilantro if desired.

Nutritional Value per serving:

- Calories: 350 , Protein: 15g
- Carbohydrates: 60g, Fat: 5g

Cooking Time: 30 minutes

Serving: 4

Edamame Salad with Miso Dressing

Ingredients:

1 cup cooked quinoa

1 cup shelled edamame, cooked and cooled

1/2 cup chopped cucumber

1/4 cup chopped red bell pepper

1/4 cup crumbled feta cheese (optional)

For the miso dressing:

1 tablespoon white miso paste

1 tablespoon rice vinegar

1 teaspoon sesame oil

1/2 teaspoon honey

Pinch of ginger powder

Preparation:

1. In a large bowl, combine cooked quinoa, edamame, cucumber, and red bell pepper.
2. In a small bowl, mix miso paste, rice vinegar, sesame oil, honey, and ginger powder until smooth.
3. Pour in your miso dressing over the salad and toss to coat.
4. Top with crumbled feta cheese (optional) and serve.

Nutritional Value (per serving):

- Calories: 350, Fat: 10g
- Carbohydrates: 40g, Protein: 20g, Fiber: 5g

Cooking Time: 15 minutes

Vegan-Friendly Recipes:

Rainbow Veggie Bowl with Tahini Dressing

Ingredients:

1 cup cooked brown rice

1/2 cup roasted sweet potato cubes

1/2 cup steamed broccoli florets

1/2 cup chopped red bell pepper

1/4 cup chopped cucumber

1/4 cup cherry tomatoes

1/4 cup crushed walnuts (optional)

For the Tahini Dressing:

2 tablespoons tahini paste

2 teaspoons lemon juice

1 tablespoon olive oil

1 clove garlic, minced

1/4 cup water

Pinch of salt and pepper

Preparation:

1. Cook brown rice according to package instructions.

2. Roast sweet potato cubes at 400°F (200°C) for 20-25 minutes, or until tender-crisp.

3. Steam broccoli florets for 5-7 minutes, or until tender-crisp.

4. In a bowl, add cooked brown rice, roasted sweet potato, steamed

broccoli, sliced bell pepper, cucumber, and cherry tomatoes.

5. Make the Tahini Dressing: In a small jar or blender, combine tahini paste, lemon juice, olive oil, garlic, water, salt, and pepper. Blend until smooth and creamy.

6. Drizzle tahini dressing over the veggie dish and top with crumbled walnuts (optional).

Nutritional Value (per serving):

- Calories: 450, Fat: 15g
- Carbohydrates: 50g, Protein: 10g, Fiber: 10g

Cooking Time: 30 minutes

Serving: 1

Lentil Shepherd's Pie with Mashed Cauliflower

Ingredients:

For the Shepherd's Pie:

1 tablespoon olive oil

1 onion, chopped

2 cloves garlic, minced

1 carrot, chopped

1 celery stalk, chopped

1 cup green lentils, rinsed

2 cups vegetable broth

1 (14.5 oz) can of chopped tomatoes, undrained

1 teaspoon dried thyme

1/2 teaspoon dried rosemary

Salt and pepper to taste

For the Mashed Cauliflower:

1 head cauliflower, cut into florets

1/4 cup unsweetened plant-based milk

1 tablespoon nutritional yeast (optional)

Salt and pepper to taste

Preparation:

1. Preheat the oven to 375°F (190°C).
2. Warm your olive oil in a big pot over medium heat and then add onion,

garlic, carrot, and celery. Cook for 5 minutes, until softened.

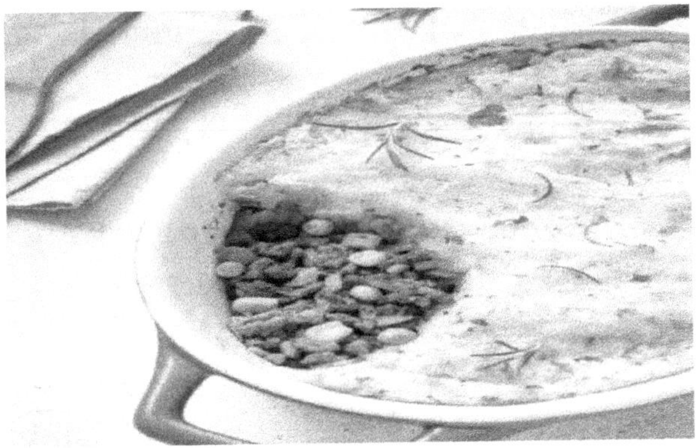

3. Stir in lentils, vegetable broth, diced tomatoes, thyme, rosemary, salt, and pepper. Bring to a boil, then decrease heat and simmer for 20-25 minutes, or until lentils are cooked.

4. While lentils simmer, cook cauliflower florets for 10-15 minutes, or until tender.

5. Mash cauliflower with plant-based milk, nutritional yeast (optional), salt, and pepper.

6. Pour the lentil mixture into a baking dish and top with mashed cauliflower then bake for 15-20 minutes or until golden brown and bubbling.

Nutritional Value (per serving):

- Calories: 400, Fat: 10g
- Carbohydrates: 55g, Protein: 18g, Fiber: 12g

Cooking Time: 45 minutes

Serving: 1

Creamy Vegan Tomato Pasta with Spinach and Roasted Vegetables

Ingredients:

1 cup cooked whole-wheat pasta

One (14.5 oz) can of chopped tomatoes, undrained

1/2 cup unsweetened plant-based milk

2 cloves garlic, minced

1/4 cup chopped fresh basil

1 tablespoon olive oil

1/2 cup chopped broccoli florets

1/2 cup cherry tomatoes

Salt and pepper to taste

Preparation:

1. Preheat the oven to 400°F (200°C).

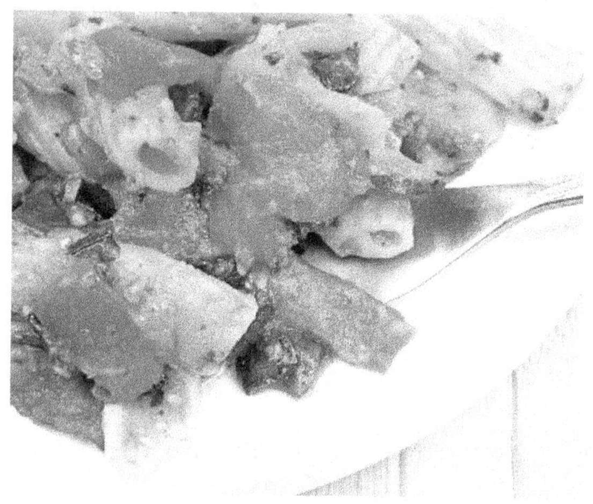

2. Toss broccoli florets and cherry tomatoes with olive oil, salt, and pepper. Spread on a baking sheet and roast for 15-20 minutes or until tender-crisp.

3. Meanwhile, cook whole-wheat pasta according to package instructions.

4. In a blender, combine chopped tomatoes, plant-based milk, garlic,

and basil. Blend until smooth and creamy.

5. Warm your tomato sauce in a saucepan over medium heat and then season with salt and pepper to taste.

6. Drain cooked pasta and combine it with the tomato sauce.

7. Serve spaghetti topped with roasted vegetables and more fresh basil (optional).

Nutritional Value (per serving):

- Calories: 400, Fat: 10g
- Carbohydrates: 60g, Protein: 15g
- Fiber: 5g

Cooking Time: 30 minutes

Serving: 1

Eggplant and Lentil Ratatouille with Brown Rice

Ingredients:

One cup brown rice, washed

1 large eggplant, diced

1 zucchini, diced

1 bell pepper, diced

1 onion, finely chopped

2 cloves garlic, minced

One can (14 oz) smashed tomatoes

One cup of dry green or brown lentils, cooked

Two tablespoons of olive oil

1 teaspoon dried thyme

1 teaspoon dried rosemary

Salt and pepper to taste

Fresh basil for garnish (optional)

Preparation:

1. In a pot, prepare brown rice according to package instructions.
2. In a big pot, warm your olive oil over medium heat, and then sauté your chopped onions and minced garlic until softened.
3. Add diced eggplant, zucchini, and bell pepper to the pot. Cook until vegetables begin to soften.
4. Stir in dried rosemary, salt, dried thyme, and pepper.

5. Add crushed tomatoes and cooked lentils to the pot. Simmer until vegetables are soft.

6. Adjust spice to taste.

7. Serve the eggplant and lentil ratatouille over a bed of cooked brown rice.

8. Decorate with fresh basil if desired.

Nutritional Value per serving:

- Calories: 380 , Protein: 18g
- Carbohydrates: 55g, Fat: 10g

Cooking Time: 40 minutes

Serving: 2 servings

Cauliflower and Chickpea Curry with Basmati Rice

Ingredients:

1 cup basmati rice, rinsed

1 head cauliflower, cut into florets

Rinsed and drained one can (15 oz) of chickpeas

1 onion, finely chopped

2 cloves garlic, minced

1 can (14 oz) coconut milk

1 tablespoon curry powder

1 teaspoon ground coriander

1 teaspoon ground cumin

1 tablespoon olive oil

Salt and pepper to taste

Fresh parsley for garnish (optional)

Preparation:

1. In a pot, prepare basmati rice according to the package instructions.

2. In a large pot, warm your olive oil over medium heat and then sauté chopped onions and minced garlic until softened.

3. Add cauliflower florets to the pot and cook for a few minutes until lightly browned.

4. Stir in curry powder, ground coriander, and ground cumin. Mix well.

5. Add chickpeas and coconut milk. Transfer to a simmer and cook until the cauliflower is tender.

6. Season with salt and pepper to taste.

7. Serve the cauliflower and chickpea curry over a bed of cooked basmati rice.

8. Garnish with fresh parsley if desired.

Nutritional Value per serving:

- Calories: 380 , Protein: 12g
- Carbohydrates: 60g, Fat: 15g

Cooking Time: 30 minutes

Serving: 2

Quinoa and Vegetable Stir-Fry with Peanut Sauce

Ingredients:

1 cup quinoa, washed

1 cup broccoli florets

1 bell pepper, sliced

1 carrot, julienned

1 cup snap peas

1/2 cup chopped green onions

1/4 cup peanuts, chopped

2 tablespoons sesame oil

2 teaspoons soy sauce (low-sodium)

1 tablespoon maple syrup

1 tablespoon rice vinegar

1 teaspoon grated ginger

1 clove garlic, minced

Salt and pepper to taste

Preparation:

1. In a saucepan, prepare quinoa according to package instructions.

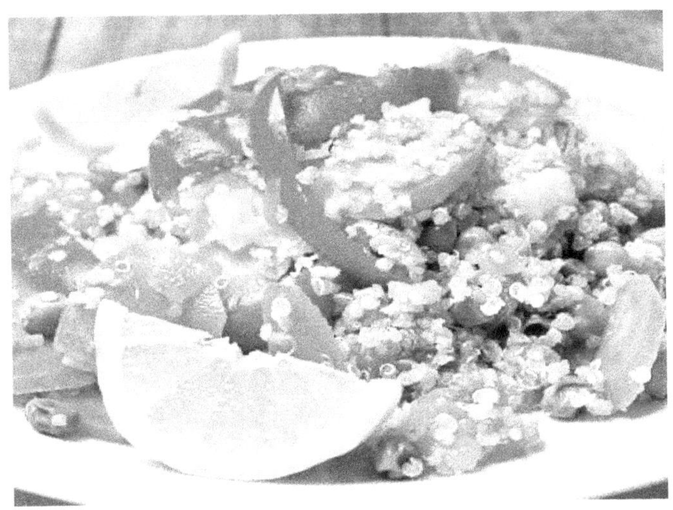

2. In a wok or large pan, warm your sesame oil over medium-high heat.

3. Stir-fry bell pepper, broccoli, carrot, and snap peas until they are crisp-tender.

4. In a small bowl, whisk together soy sauce, maple syrup, rice vinegar, grated ginger, chopped garlic, salt, and pepper.

5. Add cooked quinoa and the sauce to the wok. Mix well to coat the vegetables and quinoa.

6. Stir in chopped green onions and peanuts.

7. Cook for another 2-3 minutes until everything is cooked thoroughly.

8. Serve the quinoa and veggie stir-fry with peanut sauce.

Nutritional Value per serving:

- Calories: 400 , Protein: 15g
- Carbohydrates: 50g
- Fat: 18g

Cooking Time: 25 minutes

Serving: 2

Guacamole with Vegetable Sticks

Ingredients:

1 ripe avocado, mashed

1/4 cup chopped tomato

1 tablespoon lime juice

1/4 teaspoon minced red onion

Pinch of salt and pepper

Carrot sticks, cucumber slices, or bell pepper strips (for dipping)

Preparation:

1. Mash avocado in a bowl.

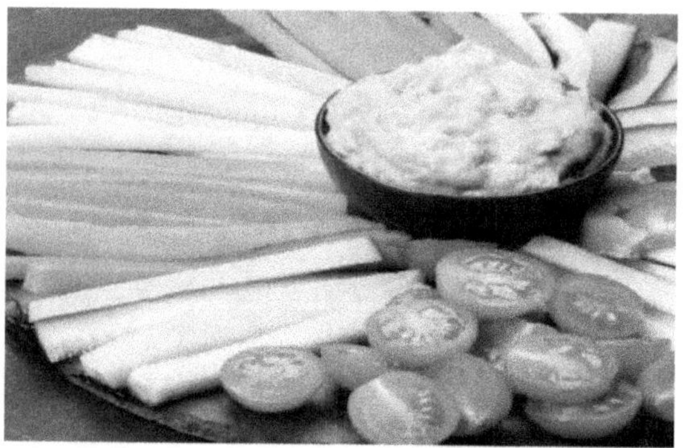

2. Stir in chopped tomato, lime juice, red onion, salt, and pepper.
3. Serve guacamole with your choice of vegetable sticks for dipping.

Nutritional Value (per serving):

- Calories: 200, Fat: 15g
- Carbohydrates: 10g, Protein: 2g
- Fiber: 5g

Preparation Time: 5 minutes

Serving: 1

Turmeric & Hummus Veggie Wraps

Ingredients:

4 whole grain or gluten-free wraps

1 cup hummus

1 cucumber, julienned

1 bell pepper, thinly sliced

1 carrot, julienned

1 tablespoon olive oil

1 teaspoon ground turmeric

Salt and pepper to taste

Fresh cilantro for garnish (optional)

Preparation:

1. Lay out the wrappers on a clean surface.

2. Spread a uniform coating of hummus on each wrap.

3. In a bowl, mix julienned cucumber, sliced bell pepper, and julienned carrot.

4. Drizzle olive oil over the vegetables and sprinkle ground turmeric, salt, and pepper. Toss to coat and then Share the veggie mixture evenly among the wraps.

5. Roll up the wraps and chop them into bite-sized pieces.

6. Garnish with fresh cilantro if desired.

Nutritional Value per serving:

- Calories: 200, Protein: 7g
- Carbohydrates: 25g, Fat: 9g

Spicy Roasted Chickpeas

Ingredients:

Rinsed and drained one can (15 oz) chickpeas

1 tablespoon olive oil

1 teaspoon ground cumin

1 teaspoon smoked paprika

1/2 teaspoon cayenne pepper (modify to taste)

1/2 teaspoon garlic powder

Salt to taste

Preparation:

1. Preheat the oven to 400°F (200°C).

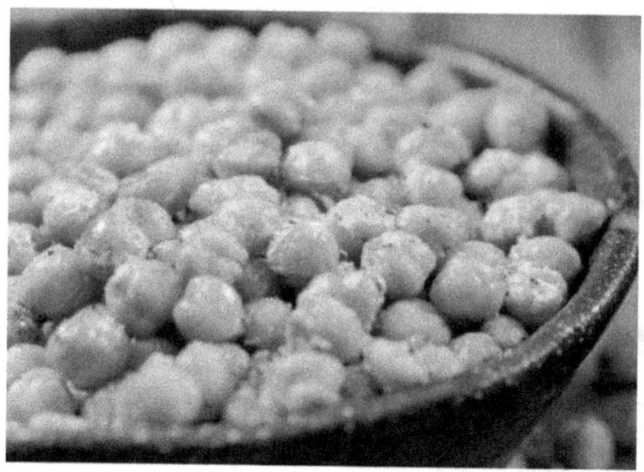

2. Pat dry the chickpeas with a clean kitchen towel to remove extra moisture.

3. In a bowl, combine chickpeas with olive oil, ground cumin, smoked paprika, cayenne pepper, garlic powder, and salt.

4. Spread the seasoned chickpeas on a baking pan in a single layer.

5. Roast in the preheated oven for 25-30 minutes or until the chickpeas are

crispy, stirring the pan halfway through, and then allow the roasted chickpeas to cool before serving.

Nutritional Value:

- Calories: 120 , Protein: 5g
- Carbohydrates: 15g, Fat: 5g

Preparation Time: 35 minutes

Serving: 4

Cottage Cheese with Pineapple and Sliced Almonds

Ingredients:

1/2 cup cottage cheese

1/4 cup chopped pineapple

1 tablespoon sliced almonds

Preparation:

1. In a bowl, combine cottage cheese, pineapple, and almonds.
2. Mix thoroughly and enjoy.

Nutritional Value (per serving):

- Calories: 180, Fat: 5g
- Carbohydrates: 10g, Protein: 15g
- Fiber: 1g

Preparation Time: 2 minutes

Serving: 1

Edamame with Sea Salt and Chili Flakes

Ingredients:

1 cup shelled edamame, frozen or fresh

1/2 teaspoon sea salt

Pinch of chili flakes (optional)

Preparation:

1. If using frozen edamame, prepare according to package instructions.
2. For fresh edamame, blanch in boiling water for 2-3 minutes, then drain and rinse with cold water.

Avocado and Tomato Salsa with Whole Grain Crackers

Ingredients:

1 ripe avocado, diced

1 cup cherry tomatoes, diced

1/4 red onion, coarsely chopped

1/4 cup cilantro, chopped Juice of 1 lime

Salt and pepper to taste

Whole grain crackers

Preparation:

1. In a bowl, combine diced avocado, diced cherry tomatoes, chopped red onion, and chopped cilantro.
2. Squeeze lime juice over the mixture and gently stir.
3. Season with salt and pepper to taste.
4. Allow the salsa to settle for a few minutes to let the flavors blend.
5. Serve the avocado and tomato salsa with whole-grain crackers.

Nutritional Value per serving:

- Calories: 200, Protein: 3g
- Carbohydrates: 20g, Fat: 12g

Preparation Time: 10 minutes

Serving: 2 servings

Kale Chips with Nutritional Yeast

Ingredients:

1 bunch kale, rinsed and dried

1 tablespoon olive oil

2 teaspoons nutritional yeast

1/2 teaspoon garlic powder

Salt to taste

Preparation:

1. Preheat the oven to 350°F (175°C).
2. Remove the stems from the kale leaves and shred them into bite-sized pieces.
3. In a bowl, combine kale pieces with olive oil, nutritional yeast, garlic powder, and salt.
4. Spread the seasoned kale on a baking pan in a single layer and then bake in the preheated oven for 10-15 minutes or until the edges are crispy.
5. Allow kale chips for some minutes to cool before serving.

Nutritional Value per serving:

- Calories: 100, Protein: 5g
- Carbohydrates: 10g, Fat: 6g

Preparation Time: 20 minutes

Serving: 2

Mango Salsa with Cucumber Slices

Ingredients:

1 ripe mango, diced

1/2 cucumber, diced

1/4 red onion, finely chopped

1 jalapeño, seeded and diced

Juice of 1 lime

2 tablespoons fresh cilantro, chopped

Salt to taste

Cucumber slices for dipping

Preparation:

1. In a bowl, add diced mango, diced cucumber, chopped red onion, diced jalapeño, lime juice, and chopped cilantro.
2. Gently whisk the ingredients together.
3. Add a little salt to the mango salsa.
4. Allow the salsa to chill in the refrigerator for at least 15 minutes.
5. Serve the mango salsa with cucumber slices for a delightful and low-calorie snack.

Nutritional Value per serving:

- Calories: 80, Protein: 1g
- Carbohydrates: 20g, Fat: 0g

Preparation Time: 15 minutes

Serving: 2

Cucumber and Hummus Bites

Ingredients:

1 large cucumber, sliced into rounds

1/2 cup hummus

Cherry tomatoes, halved

Fresh basil leaves for garnish

Olive oil for drizzling

Salt and pepper to taste

Preparation:

1. Place cucumber rounds on a serving tray.

2. Spoon a small spoonful of hummus onto each cucumber round.

3. Top with a halved cherry tomato.

4. Pour slowly olive oil over the bites and sprinkle with salt and pepper.

5. Garnish with fresh basil leaves.

6. Serve these cool nibbles for a quick and pleasant snack.

Nutritional Value per serving:

- Calories: 80 , Protein: 3g
- Carbohydrates: 8g, Fat: 5g

Preparation Time: 10 minutes

Serving: 4

Mixed Nut Trail Mix with Dried Fruits

Ingredients:

1/2 cup almonds

1/2 cup walnuts

1/4 cup pumpkin seeds

1/4 cup dried cranberries

1/4 cup dried apricots, chopped

1/4 cup dark chocolate chips (optional)

1/2 teaspoon ground cinnamon

1/4 teaspoon sea salt

Preparation:

1. In a bowl, add almonds, walnuts, pumpkin seeds, dried cranberries,

chopped dried apricots, and dark chocolate chips.

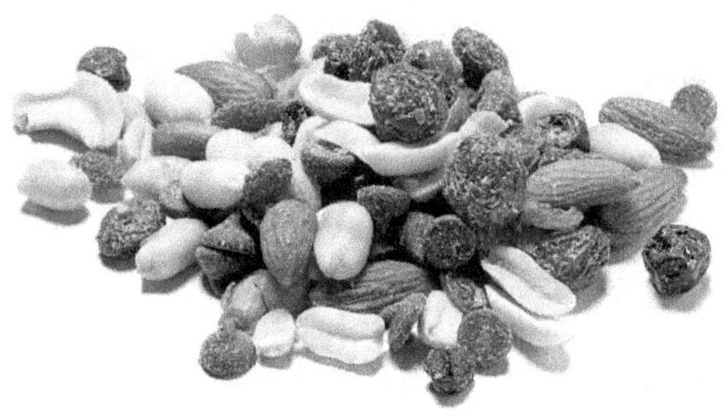

2. Sprinkle ground cinnamon and sea salt over the mixture.

3. Toss the ingredients until fully blended.

4. Portion the mixed nut trail mix into tiny snack-sized containers.

5. Enjoy this nutrient-packed trail mix as a handy and savory snack.

Nutritional Value per serving:

- Calories: 180, Protein: 5g
- Carbohydrates: 15g, Fat: 12g

Preparation Time: 5 minutes

Serving: 4

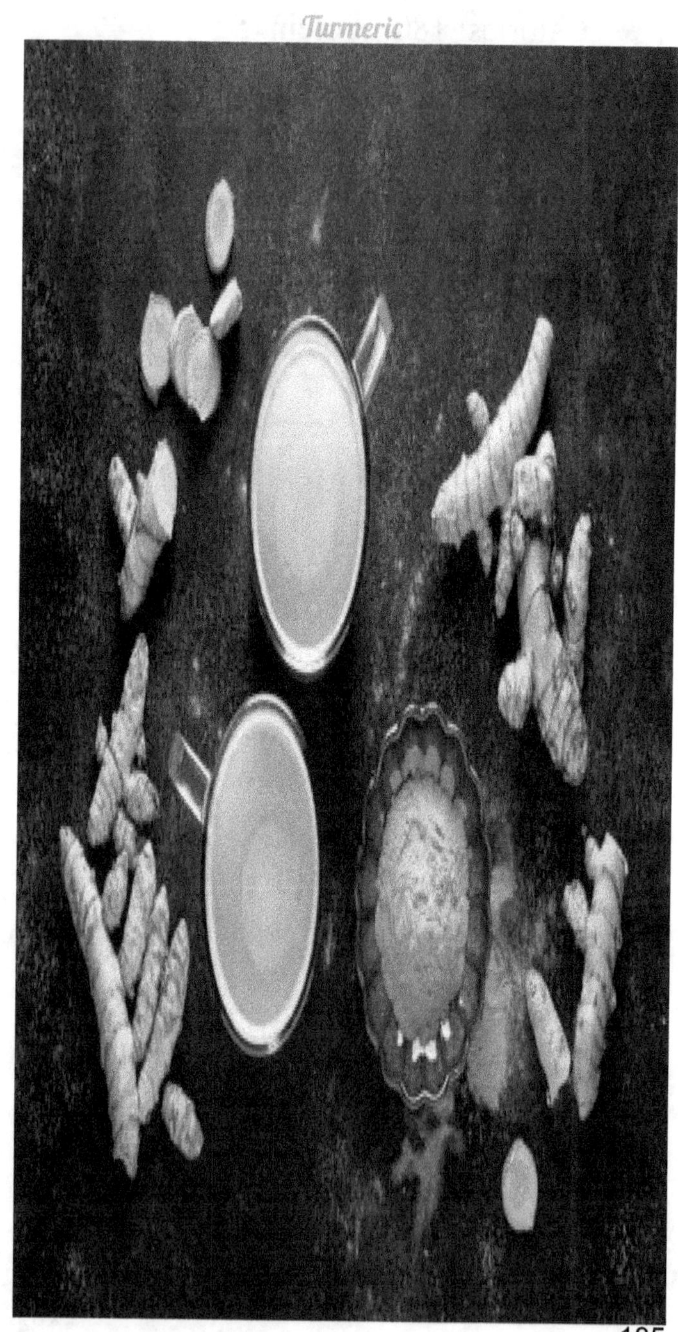

Chapter 7: Strategies To Reduce Chronic Inflammation

It is essential to promote general health and reduce the risk of chronic inflammation by implementing methods to minimize or mitigate the various factors that contribute to inflammation. Listed below are a few prevalent causes and solutions to these problems:

★ *Eating Habits:*

- Inflammatory Food Factors: A diet low in fruits and vegetables, heavy in refined sugars and saturated fats, and processed foods is one cause of inflammation.

Methods for Avoidance:

➤ Choose a diet heavy in plant-based foods, whole grains, and protein sources.

➤ Cut down on processed meals, sugary snacks, and red meat.

➤ Include more anti-inflammatory items in your diet, like nuts, seeds, fatty salmon, and olive oil.

★ *Insufficient Exercise:*

- Inflammation Factors: Inactivity is a risk factor for developing chronic inflammation.

Methods for Avoidance:

➤ Engage in regular physical activity, including aerobic workouts, strength training, and flexibility exercises.

➢ Try to achieve at least 150 minutes of moderate-intensity exercise every week.

★ *Stress Levels:*

- Contributors to Inflammation: Chronic stress can produce an inflammatory response in the body.

Methods for Avoidance:

➢ Practice stress-reducing practices such as mindfulness, meditation, deep breathing exercises, and yoga.

➢ Prioritize proper sleep to support stress management.

★ *Environmental Toxins:*

- Contributors to Inflammation: Exposure to pollution, insecticides, and other environmental poisons.

Methods for Avoidance:

- ➢ Choose organic produce when possible to reduce exposure to pesticides.
- ➢ Be careful of air quality and minimize exposure to pollutants.
- ➢ Use eco-friendly and non-toxic household items.

★ *Chronic Infections:*

- Contributors to Inflammation: Persistent infections can lead to chronic inflammation.

Methods for Avoidance:

> ➤ Practice proper hygiene to limit the risk of illnesses.
> ➤ Get inoculated against preventable diseases.
> ➤ Seek quick medical assistance for any chronic infections.

★ ***Excessive Alcohol Consumption:***

- Contributors to Inflammation: Heavy alcohol intake can contribute to inflammation and damage to organs.

Methods for Avoidance:

> ➤ Consume alcohol in moderation, if at all.

➢ Stay under prescribed limits (up to one drink per day for women and up to two drinks per day for males).

★ *Obesity:*

● Contributors to Inflammation: Excess body weight, especially visceral fat, can contribute to chronic inflammation.

Methods for Avoidance:

➢ Maintain a healthy weight through a balanced diet and regular physical activity.

➢ Focus on long-term lifestyle improvements rather than crash diets.

★ *Genetic Factors:*

- Contributors to Inflammation: Genetic predisposition may influence an individual's sensitivity to inflammation.

Avoidance Strategies:

➢ While genetics have a part, lifestyle adjustments can still assist reduce inflammation.

➢ Work with healthcare specialists to adapt methods based on genetic predispositions.

Conclusion

For coming this far congratulations on taking the first step towards a healthier and more vibrant you! Throughout this cookbook, you've explored a variety of delicious and healthy meals meant to support your body's natural anti-inflammatory response.

From building an anti-inflammatory kitchen to crafting mindful meal planning, each chapter serves as a stepping stone toward a healthier and more vibrant life. The carefully chosen recipes, meal plans, and snack ideas are not only delicious but also meant to harness the power of nutritious, nutrient-rich ingredients that reduce inflammation.

You have been armed with knowledge regarding the impact of lifestyle factors, including stress, physical activity, and sleep, on inflammation. By adopting the principles suggested in this cookbook, you have the tools to make educated decisions that transcend beyond the kitchen—choices that positively influence every part of your life.

Remember, going on the road of an anti-inflammatory diet is not about deprivation; it's about nourishment and the enjoyment of flavors. It's a path toward accepting foods that promote healing and vitality. As you appreciate the delectable recipes, let this cookbook be a companion in your journey for a healthier, more vibrant you.

May these recipes inspire you to make conscientious decisions, not merely for the sake of preventing diseases, but for the sheer joy of eating foods that love your body back. Here's to a future filled with well-being, energy, and the myriad benefits that an anti-inflammatory lifestyle delivers. Cheers to your health, happiness, and the delightful ride that lies ahead. Welcome to the realm of anti-inflammatory living — a journey that begins anew with every healthy, tasty meal.

Remember, a successful anti-inflammatory diet is a journey, not a destination. It's about implementing little, sustainable improvements into your routine and finding delight in the process of nurturing oneself.

As you continue on your path, keep these crucial insights in mind:

concentrate mostly on whole, unprocessed foods: Prioritize fruits, vegetables, whole grains, lean proteins, and healthy fats.

Explore a variety of anti-inflammatory ingredients: Experiment with meals that combine turmeric, ginger, berries, leafy greens, and fatty salmon.

Mindful eating practices: Pay attention to your hunger cues, taste your meal, and avoid distractions when eating.

Listen to your body: Pay attention to how various meals make you feel and change your diet accordingly.

Remember, this cookbook is simply a beginning point. There's a whole world of anti-inflammatory recipes waiting to be found. Embrace the opportunity to explore new flavors, cooking techniques, and ingredients. Most importantly, have fun and enjoy the wonderful path towards a healthier, happier self!

www.ingramcontent.com/pod-product-compliance
Lightning Source LLC
Chambersburg PA
CBHW050809260726
48660CB00004B/1325